Transplant Administration

Transplant Administration

Lisa Norris, MS, MBA
Managing Director and Principal, Transplant Leadership Institute LLC
San Antonio, TX, USA

WILEY Blackwell

Registered office: John Wiley & Sons, Ltd, The Atrium, Southern Gate, Chichester, West Sussex, PO19 8SQ, UK

Editorial offices: 9600 Garsington Road, Oxford OX4 2DQ, UK
The Atrium, Southern Gate, Chichester, West Sussex PO19 8SQ, UK
111 River Street, Hoboken, NJ 07030-5774, USA

For details of our global editorial offices, for customer services and for information about how to apply for permission to reuse the copyright material in this book, please see our website at www.wiley.com/wiley-blackwell

Library of Congress Cataloging-in-Publication Data

Norris, Lisa, author.
Transplant administration / Lisa Norris.
p. ; cm.
Includes bibliographical references and index.
ISBN 978-1-118-34663-1 (cloth)
I. Title.
[DNLM: 1. Tissue and Organ Procurement–organization & administration–United States. WO 660]
RD120.7
617.9′54–dc23 2013042098

A catalogue record for this book is available from the British Library.

Wiley also publishes its books in a variety of electronic formats. Some content that appears in print may not be available in electronic books.

Cover images: From left to right – iStock file #345106 © Hohenhaus, iStock file #18034935 © uchar, iStock file #21237619 © Squaredpixels, iStock file #5002422 © Platinus. Background image iStock #1224549 © Nikada.
Cover design by Meaden Creative

Set in 9.5/13pt Meridien by Aptara Inc., New Delhi, India
Printed and bound in Malaysia by Vivar Printing Sdn Bhd

1 2014

Contents

List of Contributors

Kenneth Andreoni, MD, is a pediatric and adult multi-organ abdominal transplant surgeon at University of Florida and Shands Hospital. He is the current surgical director of kidney and pancreas transplantation, and participates in liver transplantation. His faculty academic appointments were previously at The Ohio State University and the Universities of North Carolina and Arizona. He completed a transplant surgical fellowship at The Ohio State University, general surgery training and transplant research fellowship at Johns Hopkins University Hospital, and medical school training at Yale School of Medicine. Ken has been involved in UNOS National Committees for over 10 years and is currently the President of UNOS. Ken was the founding chair of the UNOS Kidney Paired Donation, prior chair of the Kidney Committee and involved in the development of a deceased kidney graft Donor Risk Index. He has basic science publications in cytomegalovirus drug therapies, ischemia-reperfusion injury, and many clinical transplant publications. Ken is currently involved in developing a local pediatric transition healthcare program with focus on transition of pediatric kidney transplant recipients to adult healthcare.

Marguerite Brown, BSN, MSN, has over 30 years experience in the field of transplantation and has served in a variety of roles including the direct care of patients, procurement of donor organs, and administrative responsibilities as a director for transplant services in multi-organ programs located in academic hospital settings. She spent the majority of her career at Stanford University Medical Center culminating in her position as the Administrative Director for Transplant Services. Marguerite currently provides interim transplant management services and has been a quality consultant for centers engaged in systems improvement agreements with CMS. She earned her Bachelor's degree in nursing from Columbia University and her Master's degree as a Cardiovascular Clinical Nurse Specialist at UCSF. She has published articles and book chapters on organ donor management and procurement of the heart and lungs.

Lauren E. Kearns, MSN, RN-BC, has over 35 years of experience in nursing, which includes 20 years experience in healthcare management and the field of transplantation. She is currently the Director of Transplant Services for the University of North Carolina Health Care System, in Chapel Hill, North Carolina. Lauren serves on the Board of Directors for Carolina Donor Services, and NC Donate Life. Lauren received her Bachelor's Degree in Nursing from the University of Illinois and earned her Master's Degree in Nursing from the University of North Carolina, Chapel Hill, specializing in Health Care Systems/Informatics. Lauren earned a Post-Master's Certificate in Nursing Education and is currently enrolled in the Doctoral Program for Information Science at UNC-CH School of Information and Library Science. She has maintained current certification with the American Nurses Credentialing Center (ANCC) in Nursing Informatics since 2004. Lauren is an Adjunct Professor–Course Coordinator for Healthcare Informatics at the University of North Carolina–Chapel Hill (UNC-CH) School of Nursing.

Lisa Norris, MS, MBA, has over 20 years of experience in healthcare management and has over 16 years of experience in the field of transplantation. She is currently the Managing Director and Principal of Transplant Leadership Institute LLC, the leading recruitment and search firm serving the fields of transplantation and organ procurement. She has served as a transplant administrator at a number of prestigious institutions: CHRISTUS Transplant Institute in San Antonio, Texas; UNC Center for Transplant Care at the University of North Carolina Health Care System in Chapel Hill, North Carolina; University of Maryland Medical System in Baltimore, Maryland; and the University of Colorado Hospital in Denver, Colorado. She has been a Region 8 administrator on the UNOS Transplant Administrator's Committee and has held various board positions with other transplant-related organizations. Lisa is a graduate of the University of Colorado, Boulder, and earned a MS degree from Northeastern University and a MBA from the Leeds School of Business at the University of Colorado.

Ciara J. Samana, MSPH, served as a policy analyst and the Liaison to the Kidney Transplantation Committee for the United Network for Organ Sharing. Previous work includes development of a new, national kidney allocation system for the Organ Procurement and Transplantation Network (OPTN). Prior to joining UNOS, Ms. Samana was an associate at the Lewin Group where she focused on evidence-based analyses for clinical topics of national importance for the Agency for Healthcare Research and Quality and analysis of the clinical, economic and market value of *in vitro* diagnostics for a large medical devices industry association. Ms. Samana's experience includes systematic evidence analysis, research on national access to pediatric subspecialists, and the contribution of non-physician providers to the healthcare workforce at the Cecil G. Sheps Center for Health Services Research. Ms. Samana also has developed educational modules on patient informed consent policy and HIV testing for the National Center for Ethics in Healthcare at the Veterans Administration in Washington, DC. In addition to health services research and policy analysis, Ms. Samana has worked as a pediatric oncology researcher at St. Jude Children's Research Hospital in Memphis, Tennessee, and a clinic director for a school-based health clinic in Knoxville, Tennessee. Ms. Samana completed her undergraduate degree in biomedical ethics and biology at the University of Tennessee and a Master of Science in Public Health in health policy and administration at the University of North Carolina at Chapel Hill.

Mindy Scharlin, MPH, has over 25 years of experience in the healthcare field and over 20 years of experience in field of organ and bone marrow transplantation. Currently she holds the position of Assistant Director, Transplant and Specialty Services Contracting for Stanford Hospital and Clinics and Lucile Packard Children's Hospital at Stanford in Northern California. Prior to this position, she was a Senior Contract Manager for Kaiser Foundation Hospitals and Health Plan in Oakland, California. She also was the Interim Director of Managed Care at California Pacific Medical Center in San Francisco, California. Ms. Scharlin was a member of the faculty for the Transplant Growth and Management Collaborative through Health Resources Services Administration and currently sits on the Products and Services Committee for the National Comprehensive Cancer Network. Ms. Scharlin is a graduate of the University of Massachusetts–Amherst and earned a MPH from the University of California at Berkeley in Policy and Administration.

Preface

Transplantation as a field of medicine is a fairly new one with most of the major developments occurring within the past 40 years. As barriers to organ rejection were overcome with new immunosuppressive drugs, transplant programs began to form with surgeons, physicians, and nurses coming together to clinically manage patients.

Professional organizations and governmental regulation grew in parallel to the developing field of transplantation. With the regulatory and organizational complexity of the field expanding, administrative tasks became excessively burdensome for physicians and clinical staff. At this time, most transplant centers were within academic medical centers, therefore the surgery division managers took responsibility over all transplant administrative activity. The major tasks focused on billing, collections, budgeting, personnel management, and CMS program submissions. With the advent of managed care, increased regulatory scrutiny, and computerized medical records and data management, the scope of the division manager grew exponentially and the position of transplant administrator was created which encompassed both the cardiothoracic and abdominal transplant programs. A variety of other roles were created to support all the functions necessary to operate the program: financial coordinators, database administrators, financial analysts, contracting specialists, operations managers, and others. Managing this complexity combined with understanding the unique aspects of transplantation is integral to the success of any transplant program.

Transplant Administration is the first book to focus exclusively on the business aspects of transplantation. It is intended to be a resource for anyone wanting to gain an in-depth understanding of this complex field: senior hospital leaders, seasoned and/or novice transplant administrators, physicians, reimbursement professionals, managed care staff, or clinical staff. The goal of this book is to provide the reader with practical and detailed guidance in leading the transplant enterprise. The chapters outline the various business disciplines that are necessary to master with an emphasis on how they relate specifically to the field of transplantation. Content is based on experience, observation of successful transplant programs, and a survey of the published literature. Ideas, suggestions, examples, and tools are also provided that can be immediately put to use.

Book Overview

Chapter 1 focuses on the history of organ allocation, the creation of the United Network for Organ Sharing, and how transplant oversight and policy developed. The current state of organ allocation in the United States is explained detailing upcoming changes in allocation policy.

Chapter 2 describes the various organizational structures of transplant programs and their advantages and disadvantages with special emphasis on the growing trend of transplant institutes.

Chapter 3 concerns the management of transplant human resources from planning the workforce to recruitment and retention of these valuable and highly specialized personnel. A discussion of compensation and medical directorships is of particular interest.

Chapter 4 explores the various issues of the transplant clinical enterprise that affect the efficiency and profitability of the transplant program. These issues range from increasing the efficiency of evaluation to appropriate documentation and billing in transplant clinic.

Chapter 5 is a comprehensive review of the history and development of regulatory oversight of transplant programs and its current state. The emphasis of this chapter is on ensuring compliance within the program with an explanation of how a program can navigate the consequences of not achieving compliance.

Chapter 6 covers the financial aspects of transplantation which are unique within healthcare due to the way Medicare reimburses pre-transplant activity through the Medicare cost report. The steps to ensure accurate and complete capture of all costs are explained in detail, as well as monitoring financial performance and profitability.

Chapter 7 offers practical explanation and advice on transplant managed care contracting. The reader is taken through the steps of this process, how managed care organizations (MCO) operate, contracting basics, and the strategies that lead to a successful partnership between the MCO and the transplant program.

Chapter 8 is focused on quality and performance improvement of transplant programs and how this has become a focal point for regulatory agencies. The chapter explains how to form a quality and performance improvement program, what the regulators are looking for and how to manage any real or potential adverse events.

Chapter 9 deals with the data requirements of a transplant program and how they are developed and managed. The history of the Scientific

Registry of Transplant Recipients is discussed along with how data requirements shape the operations and viability of programs.

Chapter 10 examines the importance of establishing strategic direction for the transplant enterprise and how that influences organizational structure, marketing, profitability, and future success.

Chapter 11 presents an overview of leading and managing a transplant program, the difference between the two, and the leadership skill sets that must be mastered. Also covered is succession planning and why it is important for a thriving transplant enterprise.

Online tools are also provided with this book which can be found at www.wiley.com/go/norris/transplantadmin

Lisa Norris

Acknowledgments

I have recognized the need for a book on the business of transplantation for many years and hoped that one of my colleagues would take on the task. However, with the field of transplantation in such flux and change, I realized that a book should be published now more than ever. As I started on this journey, I received much encouragement and support from my business colleague, Frank Greaney. I am grateful for his insight and patience. Many thanks to my friends at the Cleveland Clinic and to Art Thomson for his enormous help with this project and his review of the drafts of this manuscript.

Of course, I want to acknowledge my contributors who have spent countless hours writing and editing their work for this book: Kenneth Andreoni, Ciara Samana, Mindy Scharlin, Marguerite Brown, and Lauren E. Kearns. I greatly appreciate their wisdom and expertise—without their contributions, this book would not be complete.

I also want to thank the publishing professionals at Wiley Blackwell, particularly my Editor, Thomas Hartman, who adeptly guided me through the publishing process with sage advice and assistance, and Julie Elliott, my Development Editor.

Last, but not least, I want to thank the many transplant professionals with whom I have had the privilege to work with and know during the past 20 years. The learning and knowledge that I have gained as a result of this network of professional colleagues cannot be measured.

About the Companion Website

This book is accompanied by a companion website:

www.wiley.com/go/norris/transplantadmin

The website includes the online tools:

- Admin policies
- Clinical policies
- Kidney policies
- Other organ policies
- Web content forms

CHAPTER 1
Organ Allocation: NOTA, the OPTN, and Policy Development

Kenneth Andreoni[1] *and Ciara Samana*[2]
[1]University of Florida, Gainesville, FL, USA
[2]United Network for Organ Sharing, Richmond, VA, USA

The history: why did deceased donor allocation begin?

Successful kidney transplantation began in 1954 between identical twin brothers at Peter Bent Brigham Hospital. In 1958, immunosuppression was successfully used for renal transplants in fraternal twins. Non-twin siblings were transplanted in 1960 and then non-siblings in 1961. The year 1962 saw the first successful transplant using a deceased donor kidney allograft with the introduction of azathioprine. The Uniform Anatomical Gift Act allowed those aged 18 and over to donate their organs upon death in 1968. The year 1972 saw the discovery of cyclosporine, with its introduction to patient use in 1983. With the introduction of cyclosporine, the early success due to improved acute rejection rates in deceased donor transplantation was dramatic, and the modern era of solid organ transplantation began and expanded to other extra-renal organs.

In the early and mid-1960s, as individual transplant centers originated and developed their associated hospital-centered organ procurement organizations (OPOs), there was a very high rate of early severe rejection and graft loss in deceased donor kidney transplants. The early transplant pioneers in this pre-cyclosporine era understood that they could not easily overcome the immunological barriers of greatly mismatched organs. The odds of finding well-matched organs for their small patient lists with their few local donors were scant. They saw success with better genetically or HLA (human leukocyte antigen)-matched living donor organs and attempted to extend this to deceased donor transplantation by joining together with other transplant centers and their local OPOs to better the odds of their patients finding well-matched deceased donor organs. David Hume and Bernard Amos began the effort as SEROPP, the South-Eastern Regional Organ Procurement Program. This effort expanded to eight

Transplant Administration, First Edition. Edited by Lisa Norris.

Companion website: www.wiley.com/go/norris/transplantadmin

transplant centers in the Southeast and became SEOPF, the Southeastern Organ Procurement Foundation. Soon, other adjacent centers sought membership in SEOPF, and this membership organization began to grow. SEOPF developed the Kidney Center that assisted with deceased donor kidney matching 24 hours a day. Eventually, this was renamed the United Network for Organ Sharing, UNOS. As government regulation became formal through the development of the National Organ Transplant Act (NOTA), UNOS separated from SEOPF as a not-for-profit organization; so it could apply for the Organ Procurement Transplantation Network (OPTN) and Scientific Registry for Transplant Recipients (SRTR) contracts created in NOTA and administered by the Health Resources and Services Administration (HRSA) of the US Department of Health and Human Services (HHS). UNOS remains a membership organization consisting of transplant centers, OPOs, donor families, organ recipients and candidates, prior living donors, and others interested in organ transplantation. The Kidney Center celebrated 30 years of continuous operation in 2012 [1].

Organ allocation

Organ allocation in the United States is governed by a complex, multifaceted set of policies. These policies are used to program the national allocation system by which candidates are identified and prioritized for organ offers. There are many players in the field of organ transplantation, and the field is highly regulated at multiple levels. At the federal level, NOTA and OPTN Final Rule set the requirements for policy development. These requirements are executed by the OPTN Board of Directors and its 20 committees (Figure 1.1) in the development of policies. Policies are developed collaboratively within the committee and Board structure, with input and comment provided by the transplant community, general public, and HRSA representation. The regulatory requirements,

- Ad hoc Disease Transmission Advisory
- Ad hoc International Relations
- Ethics
- Executive
- Finance
- Histocompatibility
- Kidney Transplantation
- Liver and Intestinal Organ Transplantation
- Living Donor
- Membership and Professional Standards
- Minority Affairs
- Operations and Safety
- OPO
- Pancreas Transplantation
- Patient Affairs
- Pediatric Transplantation
- Policy Oversight
- Thoracic Organ Transplantation
- Transplant Administrators
- Transplant Coordinators

Figure 1.1 OPTN/UNOS Committees.

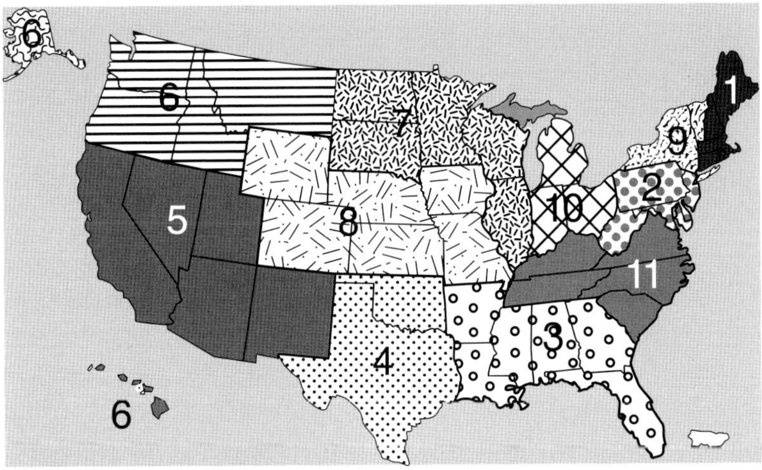

Figure 1.2 The UNOS regions.

applicable ethical frameworks, and policy development process are described in greater detail later in the chapter.

Organ allocation for kidney, pancreas, and liver grafts has traditionally followed the concept of "local, then regional, then national" allocation. The local unit of allocation generally involves the center(s) served by an individual OPO. The country has traditionally been divided into 11 regions as seen in Figure 1.2. The regions are based mainly from historic sharing arrangements. Heart and lung allocation has transitioned to a concentric circle model centered on the location of the donor hospital. The zones include the transplant hospitals that are 500, 1000, 1500, and 2500 nautical miles from the donor hospital. The remaining chapter discusses the regulatory and ethical frameworks that guide the development of organ allocation policies.

Regulations governing organ transplantation

National Organ Transplant Act (NOTA)

The NOTA was passed in 1984 when the Congress recognized the need for a transplantation network. NOTA is the regulation that established the OPTN and the SRTR. NOTA called for the OPTN and SRTR contracts to be operated by a private, non-profit organization(s) under federal contract.

The OPTN is a unique public–private partnership that links all of the professionals involved in the donation and transplantation system. The primary goals of the OPTN are to

- increase the effectiveness and efficiency of organ sharing and equity in the national system of organ allocation;
- increase the supply of donated organs available for transplantation.

The UNOS, based in Richmond, Virginia, administers the OPTN contract. The SRTR contract is administered by the Chronic Disease Research Group of the Minneapolis Medical Research Foundation. The HRSA of the US Department of HHS is the issuing agency for both contracts.

The OPTN acts through its Board of Directors. The current UNOS Board also presently serves as the OPTN Board of Directors, with the addition of HRSA representatives to complete the OPTN Board. Board members, chosen through an open, comprehensive nomination process, bring a wealth of commitment and technical knowledge to guide the OPTN in establishing and maintaining policies and procedures for the field of transplantation [2].

Organ Procurement and Transplantation Network (OPTN) Final Rule

Effective March 16, 2000, the Department of HHS implemented a Final Rule establishing a regulatory framework for the structure and operations of the OPTN. Under the terms of the Final Rule, policies intended to be binding upon OPTN members are developed through the OPTN Committees and Board of Directors and then submitted to the Secretary of HHS for final approval.

Among other items, the OPTN Final Rule addresses the organization of the OPTN, membership, policies, listing requirements, organ procurement, identification of recipients, allocation of organs, designated transplant program requirements, and reporting requirements.

With regard to allocation of organs, the Final Rule has requirements for policy development. Allocation policies shall

- "be based on sound medical judgment;
- preserve the ability of a transplant program to decline an offer of an organ or not to use the organ for the potential recipient . . . ;
- be specific for each organ type or combination of organ types to be transplanted into a transplant candidate;
- be designed to avoid wasting organs, to avoid futile transplants, to promote patient access to transplantation, and to promote the efficient management of organ placement;
- be reviewed periodically and revised as appropriate;
- include appropriate procedures to promote and review compliance including, to the extent appropriate, prospective and retrospective reviews of each transplant program's application of the policies to patients listed or proposed to be listed at the program;
- not be based on the candidate's place of residence or place of listing, except to the extent required [by points 1–5 above]" [3].

Responsibilities of OPTN

The OPTN helps ensure the success and efficiency of the US organ transplant system. OPTN responsibilities include

- facilitating the organ matching and placement process through the use of the computer system and a fully staffed Organ Center operating 24 hours a day;
- developing consensus-based policies and procedures for organ recovery, distribution (allocation), and transportation;
- collecting and managing scientific data about organ donation and transplantation;
- providing data to the government, the public, students, researchers, and the Scientific Registry of Transplant Recipients, for use in the ongoing quest for improvement in the field of solid organ allocation and transplantation;
- developing and maintaining a secure Web-based computer system, which maintains the nation's organ transplant waiting list and recipient/donor organ characteristics (UNET^{SM} and DonorNet^{SM});
- providing professional and public education about donation and transplantation, the activities of the OPTN, and the critical need for donation [4].

Under federal law, all US transplant centers and OPOs must be members of the OPTN to receive any funds through Medicare. Other members of the OPTN include independent histocompatibility laboratories involved in organ transplantation; relevant medical, scientific, and professional organizations; relevant voluntary health and patient advocacy organizations; and members of the general public with a particular interest in donation and/or transplantation.

Responsibilities of the Scientific Registry of Transplant Recipients

The Scientific Registry of Transplant Recipients is a national database of statistics related to solid organ transplantation—kidney, liver, pancreas, intestine, heart, and lung. The SRTR contract was administered by UNOS until 2000, then the Arbor Research Collaborative for Health with the University of Michigan until 2010, and currently by Chronic Disease Research Group of the Minneapolis Medical Research Foundation.

The registry covers the full range of transplant activity, from organ donation and waiting list candidates to transplant recipients and survival statistics. Its purpose is to

- support the development of sound policy;
- encourage research on issues of importance to the transplant community;
- facilitate responsible analysis of transplant programs and OPOs.

Data in the registry are collected by the OPTN from transplant hospitals and OPOs across the country. The SRTR supplements this information by using the Social Security Master Death Data Base and Medicare database for potential re-initiation of renal replacement therapy via dialysis [5]. SRTR data will be discussed further in Chapter 9.

Ethical frameworks used in organ allocation policy development

In 1994, the OPTN/UNOS Board of Directors approved a set of guidelines for creating equitable organ allocation policies. The statement describes how organ allocation policies should balance the principles of utility (i.e., the net medical benefit to all transplant patients as a group) and justice (i.e., equity and distribution of the benefits and burdens among all transplant patients) [6].

The OPTN policy for equitable organ allocation *strikes a balance* among the following principles. The policy must

1. enhance the overall availability of transplantable organs;
2. allocate organs based on medical criteria, striving to give equal consideration to medical utility (i.e., *net* medical benefit to all transplant patients as a group) and justice (i.e., equity in distribution of the benefits and burdens among all transplant patients);
3. provide transplant candidates reasonable opportunities to be considered for organ offers within comparable time periods, taking into consideration similarities and dissimilarities in medical circumstances as well as technical and logistical factors in organ distribution;
4. respect autonomy of persons.

The goal of the OPTN organ allocation system is to achieve, *in balance with one another*, the following objectives:

1. Maximize the availability of transplantable organs by
   - **a** promoting consent for donation;
   - **b** enhancing procurement efficiency;
   - **c** minimizing organ discards;
   - **d** promoting efficiency in organ distribution and allocation.
2. Maximize patient and graft survival.
3. Minimize disparities in consistently measured waiting times until an offer of an organ for transplantation is made among patients with similar or comparable medical/demographic characteristics. (At the

present time, there are no waiting list criteria; therefore, commencement of waiting time varies among patients.)

4 Minimize deaths while waiting for a transplant.
5 Maximize opportunity for patients with biological or medical disadvantages to receive a transplant.
6 Minimize effects related to geography.
7 Allow convenient access to transplantation.
8 Minimize overall transplantation related costs.
9 Provide for flexibility in policy making.
10 Provide for accountability and public trust.

Policy development process

OPTN/UNOS strives to develop policies that are based on the best available evidence and are consensus driven. The field of organ transplantation depends on the input and collaboration of many people and organizations. It is vital to ensure that all interested parties are given a voice and an opportunity to provide input into the policy development process. The following describes how the process incorporates this input along with evidence analyses in policy development, which can be seen in Figure 1.3.

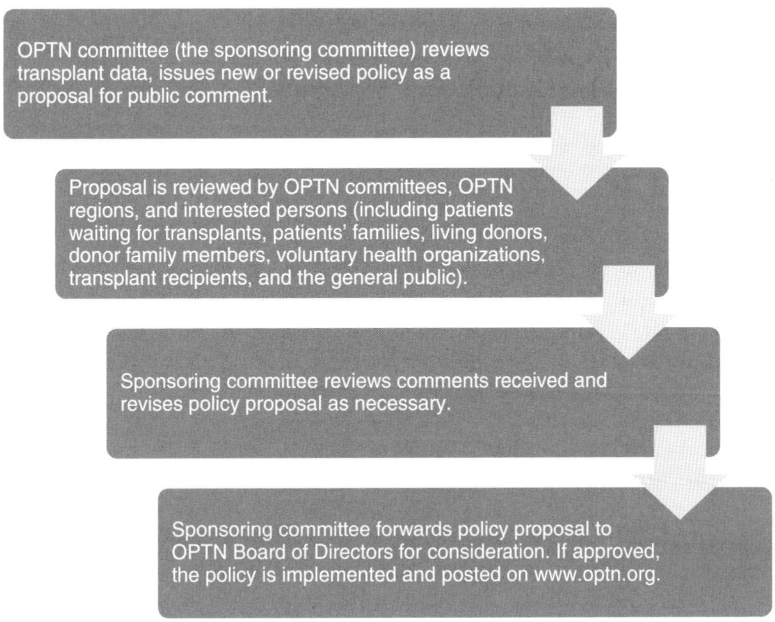

Figure 1.3 OPTN Policy development process.

The OPTN Board of Directors sets objectives for the network through a strategic plan. OPTN Committees work to meet these objectives by identifying problems within the transplant system that could be addressed through OPTN policy. Changes in policy may have different effects on individuals within the OPTN, depending on the role that each plays. Therefore, committees assess policy approaches from multiple perspectives (e.g., transplant candidate, transplant physician/surgeon, transplant coordinator, etc.). Committees also assess policy as it relates to patient safety, outcomes (e.g., patient and graft survival), and overall equity and efficiency of the allocation system. Based on the overall assessment of the full complement of policy approaches, the committee may select one approach to distribute for public comment as a policy proposal.

During the public comment period (which generally lasts between 45 and 90 days), members of OPTN/UNOS Committees, regions, and the general public are able to provide feedback on the policy proposal. Regional councilors directly advise the Board of Directors on regional discussions and votes pertaining to policy issues.

Following the public comment period, the sponsoring committee is responsible for reviewing and responding to comments provided during the review period. The committee may conduct additional analyses of the evidence before determining whether or not to submit the policy proposal to the OPTN/UNOS Board of Directors. Final proposals generally include communication and education plans, evaluation and monitoring plans, and descriptions of any automated solutions that may be necessary to the computer algorithm that matches donors and potential recipients called UNet^{sm}. The purpose of these plans is to clearly describe the resources and efforts necessary to successfully implement the policy proposal.

Once submitted, the OPTN/UNOS Board of Directors considers the policy proposal in its entirety. After discussion, the Board decides whether the policy proposal should be implemented, returned to committee for further analysis, or not implemented. On rare occasions, the Board may propose amendments to the proposal to address new or unresolved concerns. If the policy is approved for implementation, the sponsoring committee takes steps to notify the membership through an OPTN Policy Notice and may provide additional education opportunities if the proposal has a wide-reaching impact or requires major procedural changes at member institutions.

All substantial policy proposals affecting membership in OPTN/UNOS or organ allocation are distributed for public comment prior to adoption to the Board of Directors. Exceptions may be made in cases where the proposal addresses an immediate patient safety need.

Current organ allocation policies

Deceased donor kidney allocation

The current system has been in place for over 25 years, with relatively minor changes by various Kidney Committees. As immunosuppression has matured, the points used to allocate kidneys have changed dramatically. Initially, "matching" played the major role in allocation with each of the six HLAs used for allocation purposes given two points for each match between the candidate and recipient. The HLA antigens historically include A, B and DR, with each person having two alleles of each, so sometimes written as HLA – A1, A2, B1, B2, DR1 and DR2. A total of 12 points was therefore possible for a "6 antigen match" or "zero-mismatch" between the donor and recipient candidate. Time was given one point for a year of waiting (time placed on the list), and if a candidate was highly sensitized with a panel reactive antibody (PRA) level 80 percent or higher, they received another 4 points. These highly sensitized patients were very difficult to transplant until very recently with advanced solid-phase testing for specific alloantibodies. As immunosuppression improved, HLA-B points were removed when it was shown that HLA-B matching was of very marginal benefit in regard to preventing rejection and was disproportionately unfair due to the difference in HLA-B antigens in African Americans versus non-African Americans. Later, HLA-A points were removed, leaving the current policy of one point for each HLA-DR locus match. Today, patients receive a maximum of two points for HLA-DR matching. Patients still receive 4 points if their calculated PRA (CPRA) is $\geq$80%, but the CPRA value is now established by a calculator found on the OPTN website based on donor population genetics, and is a true estimate of the chance of a candidate finding a donor who does not have unacceptable antigens based on sophisticated alloantibody determination in the candidates. *Time is the major determinate of points over the last several years in most areas of the country.* Waiting time is still measured from the time the candidate is placed on the waiting list at a transplant center, which can be anytime after starting dialysis, or with a calculated GFR of 20 mg/dL or less.

In 2009, the mandatory sharing rules for zero-mismatch (0-mm) allocation changed to decrease the organs sent long distances to unsensitized patients in order to decrease the very complicated "payback" system across the country, as well as to improve graft function overall since the payback system was resulting in an overall net loss of allograft function. This change decreased the net sharing of kidneys for 0-mm allocation by almost 50% within the first year and has allowed OPOs to pay back their kidney debts and also engage in simultaneous kidney–pancreas (SKP) transplantation (an option that was not available to transplant programs served by OPOs with excessive debt levels).

"Pediatric Share 35" allocation went into practice in September, 2005. This policy gives pediatric candidates, defined as those placed on the waiting list prior to their eighteenth birthday, high priority for kidneys from local donors under the age of 35 years. These pediatric recipients follow those candidates for multiorgan transplant (pancreas–kidney, liver–kidney or heart–kidney most commonly), and some of the very highly sensitized adults. Overall around the country, most centers have had their time to transplantation for their pediatric candidates decrease dramatically. This has resulted in some areas seeing significant decreases in living donor pediatric transplantation [7].

The summary of the deceased donor allocation system can be found on the OPTN website at http://optn.transplant.hrsa.gov/PoliciesandBylaws2/policies/pdfs/policy_7.pdf.

Any changes in policies will be displayed for public comment in this area, and up-to-date policy language will always appear on this site. In June 2013, the OPTN/UNOS Board of Directors approved a proposal to completely overhaul the national kidney allocation system. Implementation of the new system is anticipated to occur by the end of 2014. The new system is hoped to provide better access to kidney transplantation for all groups of candidates while seeking to improve outcomes for kidney transplant recipients, increase the years recipients may have a functioning transplant and increase utilization of available kidneys.

In summary, deceased donor kidney allocation goes through the following categories below with points allocated within the categories as discussed earlier (Time, PRA, HLA-DR matching). For a detailed list, see http://optn.transplant.hrsa.gov/SharedContentDocuments/Kidney_Appendix_A.pdf.

For simplicity, "payback" sharing is not shown in the short summary.

For the Donors ≤35 (all SCD):

0-mm allocation (ABO identical, then compatible only for 0 to B, Pediatric then Adults, Local then Regional then National)
Prior Living Donor in local OPO
CPRA > 80; Local
Pediatric Local
Adult Local
Regional; CPRA > 80, then <80
National; CPRA > 80, then <80

For Standard Criteria Donors >35:

0-mm allocation (ABO identical, then compatible only for 0 to B, Pediatric then Adults, Local then Regional then National)
Prior Living Donor in local OPO
All Local

Regional
National
For Donation after Cardiac Death (DCD) Donors ≤35 years old:
0-mm local
Prior Living Donor in local OPO
Local highest scoring high CPRA
Local Pediatrics
All Local
Regional; CPRA >80, then <80
National; CPRA >80, then <80
For Extended Criteria Donors:
0-mm Local, Regional, National
Local only by waiting time points
Regional only by waiting time points
National only by waiting time points

The Kidney Committee's review of allocation options and likely new policy changes that are about to be released for public comment in the fall of 2012 are summarized at http://optn.transplant.hrsa.gov/kars.asp.

As of September 2012, the most likely changes being discussed for revision to Kidney Allocation policies are as follows:

1 Waiting time starting from the time of onset of chronic dialysis or listing at a transplant center with a GFR ≤ 20 mL/min.
2 Quality of kidney allograft estimated by a continuous kidney donor profile index (KDPI) [8] and no longer divided into standard criteria donor (SCD) and extended criteria donor (ECD).
3 ECD category likely to be replaced by KDPI > 85% (estimated shortest survival 15% of donor organs).
4 CPRA points on a sliding scale based on actual number of allografts offered to candidates on the list due to their CPRA. This will increase the number of points greatly after CPRA over 95.
5 Wider geographical sharing outside of the local allocation unit for the most highly sensitized patients (CPRA ≥ 99%), and higher priority for local candidates with CRPA of 98%.
6 Longest 20% estimated survivable organs allotted first to candidates with the estimated longest 20% post-transplant survival.
7 No payback of shared kidney allografts.

Kidney–pancreas allocation

Just a few years ago, there was no mandated manner to allocate SKP organs. Local OPOs were given the authority to decide how they would allocate these organs: whether SKP candidates would have their own waitlist or if SPK candidates would only be eligible for kidney allocation if their wait time was competitive with the local kidney waitlist candidates. It was well accepted that candidates on the SPK waiting list, generally type I diabetics, die at a much higher rate than patients on the kidney-alone waiting list. This led the majority of OPOs around the country to give SPK candidates their separate waiting list. The new SKP allocation policy recently went into effect and made this majority practice the national policy. It is available at http://optn.transplant.hrsa.gov/PoliciesandBylaws2/policies/pdfs/policy_10.pdf.

"Each candidate registered on the KP waiting list must be diagnosed with diabetes or have pancreatic exocrine insufficiency with renal insufficiency or require the pancreas for technical reasons as part of a multiple organ transplant." For a patient to accrue waiting time on the KP waiting list, they must qualify to start gathering waiting time for a solitary kidney (policy 3.5.11.1) and fulfill one of the following: (1) on insulin with C-peptide ≤ 2 ng/mL, (2) on insulin with C-peptide >2 ng/mL and BMI less than or equal to the maximum allowable BMI (starting at 28). The BMI will be monitored and adjusted downward if more than 15% of KP candidates on the local kidney list meet the latter criteria for KP listing.

Local offers to pancreas and KP list will precede isolated kidney allocation. P/KP allocation is based off of donor age and BMI as these predict the likelihood of whole-organ versus islet utilization.

A For donors ≤50 years of age and BMI ≤ 30:
- **a** Local 0-mm CPRA ≥ 80 P or KP
- **b** Local CPRA ≥ 80 P or KP
- **c** Regional 0-mm CPRA ≥ 80 P or KP
- **d** National 0-mm CPRA ≥ 80 P or KP
- **e** Local P and KP
- **f** Regional P or KP (if local OPO offers K) CPRA ≥ 80, then <80
- **g** National P or KP (if local OPO offers K) CPRA ≥ 80, then <80
- **h** Local pancreatic islets
- **i** Regional pancreatic islets
- **j** National pancreatic islets

B For donors >50 years of age or BMI > 30:
- **a** Local 0-mm CPRA ≥ 80 P or KP
- **b** Local CPRA ≥ 80 P or KP
- **c** Regional 0-mm CPRA ≥ 80 P or KP
- **d** National 0-mm CPRA ≥ 80 P or KP
- **e** Local P and KP
- **f** Local pancreatic islets
- **g** Regional pancreatic islets
- **h** National pancreatic islets
- **i** Regional P or KP (if local OPO offers K) CPRA ≥ 80, then <80
- **j** National P or KP (if local OPO offers K) CPRA ≥ 80, then <80

Liver allocation

The model for end-stage liver disease (MELD) score has been used for liver allocation for over 10 years now. The MELD score is calculated from a candidate's total bilirubin, serum creatinine, and international normalized ratio (INR). The MELD score for liver allocation ranges from a low of 6 points (very little probability of dying from liver failure) to a set maximum of 40 points, a very ill patient who is unlikely to survive more than a week without a liver transplant. A calculator is available on the OPTN website to show you how the laboratory value changes affect the score. This MELD score was initially calculated to estimate the survival of end-stage liver disease patients who were being considered for placement of a transjugular intrahepatic portosystemic shunt (TIPS) for severe portal hypertension. It was later shown to predict mortality for those awaiting liver transplantation. The MELD score does tend to favor those with viral hepatitis compared to those with cholestatic diseases. Several modifications to the MELD score have been proposed, with the most common being an increase in MELD points for candidates with low serum sodium (hyponatremia) as these patients tend to be more ill than patients with more normal sodium levels. Some regional review boards will give more points for difficult-to-correct hyponatremic patients, though this is not currently national policy. The other major criticism of the MELD score is that it gives a large weight of points to the serum creatinine value; thus it favors patients with kidney dysfunction. This has led to many liver recipients receiving combined liver–kidney transplants. Patients who are on dialysis receive a MELD score of 20 and are therefore competitive for a liver graft in some areas of the country. Additional details for the liver allocation policy may be found at http://optn.transplant.hrsa.gov/PoliciesandBylaws2/policies/pdfs/policy_8.pdf.

In addition to the discussed "calculated MELD score" from laboratory values, there are exception points available for certain medical conditions; the most common by far is the presence of stage 2 hepatocellular carcinoma (HCC). The Milan criteria are used to describe the category of early HCC that qualifies automatically for a MELD score of 22 points: one lesion between 2 and 5 cm, or two to three lesions with the largest 3 cm or less, and the others at least 1 cm. More stringent radiological criteria have recently been made policy and are available on the OPTN website. In addition, conditions such as hepatopulmonary syndrome, portopulmonary syndrome, and certain metabolic diseases can qualify for exception points that will increase if the patient is not transplanted within 90 days as long as the candidate continues to qualify for the exception.

Only patients with acute fulminant liver failure or a failed newly transplanted liver graft can qualify for Status 1 listing, and they must requalify every 7 days. Status 1 candidates are in the first category of liver allocation, and this group is shared regionally with a local Status 1 candidate prioritized ahead of a regional candidate. The next category of regional sharing was just approved in 2012 and is the group of patients with a MELD score ≥35. It is also prioritized as local before regional, but with each point of the MELD score from 40 down to 35 (e.g., a regional candidate with a MELD score of 39 is prioritized ahead of a local candidate with a MELD score of 38). The next category is local candidates with MELD 29–34, then national liver–intestine candidate, then local MELD scores 15 to 28, then regional 15–34, and National (Status 1 then MELD scores >15). Local, regional, and national candidates with MELD scores <15 are the last three categories for allocation. Candidates with MELD scores at or above 25 must recertify every 14 days and every month for those with MELD scores 18 to 24.

Pediatric candidates are divided above and below 11 years of age and pediatric donors are likewise allocated first to age-equivalent recipients. The pediatric end-stage liver disease (PELD) measure has been more difficult to correlate with pediatric outcome, especially at the lower values.

Recent discussions at the Liver and Intestinal Organ Transplantation Committee have included a look at a change to MELD that would not only attempt to predict pre-transplant mortality, but also consider the likelihood of patient survival after transplant.

Heart allocation

The Heart Allocation System (HAS) utilizes a circular zone concept for allocation units. These five zones are concentric circles of 500 miles from the donor hospital. The degree of illness is determined by a status code. Status 1A candidates are in the hospital with an artificial circulatory assist device just placed, or one with complications. The candidate could also be on mechanical ventilation or on continuous high-dose vasopressors with continuous left ventricular monitoring. After 14 days, most patients in Status 1A who are not unstable will drop to Status 1B (mechanical devices, low-dose pressors). Status 2 contains all other active candidates [9].

Lung allocation

The Lung Allocation Score (LAS) is very dynamic and incorporates measure of urgency for transplant (risk of death without transplant) as well as post-transplant expected survival: http://optn.transplant.hrsa.gov/PoliciesandBylaws2/policies/pdfs/policy_9.pdf. There are 12 factors used to predict risk of death, and 7 used to predict post-transplant survival. The Raw Allocation Score is calculated from Transplant Benefit Score minus Waitlist Urgency Score. This number ranges from −730 to +365 days and is then normalized on a 0 to 100 scale to give an LAS. Higher scores are higher priority for allocation. The cause of lung disease is a major predictor of both pre-transplant urgency and post-transplant survival.

Staying in compliance

The Membership and Professional Standards Committee (MPSC) oversees the outcomes of the individual transplant center organ-specific programs, as well as the overall administrative and clinical adherence to OPTN policies. Organ-specific outcome reports, termed the Program Specific Reports (PSR), are published publicly on the OPTN and SRTR websites every 6 months. They include a look at five consecutive groups of 6-month patient cohorts. Thus, they span a two-and-a half-year period of time with follow-up calculations for 1- and 3-year patient and graft survival and the actual survival is risk adjusted in order to compare a center's outcomes to the national "expected outcomes." The risk-adjusted modeling is complicated and explained in detail on the SRTR website [10]. The PSR tool was began as an internal quality evaluation tool by the MPSC, but is now used by other external groups. Changes to the PSR metric is being nationally discussed at the time of this publication [11]. A PSR Consensus Conference was attended in May 2012 by many of the transplant community to detail the needs of the public for reporting outcomes, as well as discussions of better methodology to risk adjust and allowances for study protocols and treatment of particularly high-risk recipients who may be denied transplantation without PSR modifications.

The OPTN/UNOS just completed a major rewrite of the Policy Language to help the transplant membership and public more easily understand the multitude of policy amendments over decades. This rewrite clarified the language without making substantiate changes in any of the policies. It is available online [12].

References

1 http://www.seopf.org/intro.htm. Accessed October 2, 2013.
2 www.unos.org. Accessed October 2, 2013.
3 optn.transplant.hrsa.gov. Accessed October 2, 2013.
4 optn.transplant.hrsa.gov/optn/. Accessed October 2, 2013.
5 www.srtr.org. Accessed October 2, 2013.
6 UNOS Statement of Principles and Objectives of Equitable Organ Allocation. OPTN/UNOS Board of Directors. Passed June 1994.
7 Abraham EC, Wilson AC. Goebel current kidney allocation rules and their impact on a pediatric transplant center. *J Am J Transplant.* 2009;9(2):404–408.

8 Rao PS, Schaubel DE, Guidinger MK, et al. A comprehensive risk quantification score for deceased donor kidneys: the kidney donor risk index. *Transplantation*. 2009;88(2):231–236.

9 http://optn.transplant.hrsa.gov/PoliciesandBylaws2/policies/pdfs/policy_9.pdf. Accessed October 2, 2013.

10 Background and Methodology, Program Specific Reports. Scientific Registry of Transplant Recipients. http://srtr.org/csr/current/tech_notes.aspx. Accessed October 2, 2013.

11 srtr.org/cctpqs/Default.aspx. Accessed October 2, 2013.

12 Policy Management. Organ Procurement and Transplantation Network. http://optn.transplant.hrsa.gov/plainlanguage.asp. Accessed October 2, 2013.

CHAPTER 2
Organizational Structures

Lisa Norris

Transplant Leadership Institute LLC, San Antonio, TX, USA

The structure of an organization is vital to organizational effectiveness and readiness to adapt to the changing landscape of healthcare delivery. An organization can be structured in many different ways, depending on the mission, vision, and goals of the organization. The structure of an organization will determine how it executes strategy and ultimately performs. At one end of the spectrum are traditional, bureaucratic, and pyramidal organizations, in the middle are matrix and service line organizations, and at the other end of the spectrum lies the pure integrated organization (institute) where staff is completely accountable to and for their programs.

Historically, transplant programs were housed in academic medical centers and, thus, were part of the medical school organizational structure which is vertical and functional. As the complexity of programs grew to include multiorgan transplants and a multidisciplinary approach to care, other organizational structures such as matrix and service line emerged. The latest trend for transplant programs is the development of transplant institutes which, in theory, permit an autonomous, stand-alone enterprise within the larger organization. Many programs may be called institutes; however, they have not yet achieved the true structure that the name implies. This chapter discusses each type of organizational structure, the advantages and disadvantages, and how it affects program effectiveness. The decision to move to one structure or a combination of structures is based on each program's unique situation.

Functional structure

Among the numerous types of organizational structures, the functional organizational structure is the most common, particularly in academic medical centers. The functional model has a hierarchical structure and is best suited for stable environments. This structure is bureaucratic in nature

Transplant Administration, First Edition. Edited by Lisa Norris.

Companion website: www.wiley.com/go/norris/transplantadmin

and relies on rules, policies, and procedures for work processes. The span of control is narrow and favors the development of silos.

The typical functional organizational structure usually has a department head, with division chiefs in charge of the various divisions or sections. Under the sections/divisions reside both administrative and clinical functions and the corresponding staff. Under this structure, there exist many transplant programs within the organization, specifically, within the hospital, the departments of medicine, surgery, and pediatrics, each of which can be further broken down by organ [1]. Revenue for this structure is derived from clinical income, with some hospital support coming from transplant program directorships. This creates unique challenges in creating common goals and a unified vision for the transplant program.

Advantages of a functional structure:

- The chain of command is clear and vertical.
- The development of professional expertise is attained by grouping specialists together.
- It supports an academic hierarchy.
- Resources are centralized.
- Employees' career paths are clear-cut.

Drawbacks of the functional organizational structure:

- The decision-making process is cumbersome since decisions must be moved up the chain of command.
- The flow of communication and cooperation between functional departments is complicated.
- Problem resolution is slow and inefficient.
- Staff do not have a big picture view of the overall organization.
- It does not support the multidisciplinary nature of transplant.
- There is a lack of common goals between medical and surgical transplant specialists and among abdominal and thoracic specialists, in particular.
- It is not flexible in reacting to an ever-changing healthcare environment [1].

Matrix structure

Matrix organizations were developed to deal with large projects and complexity in the external environment. These organizations employ the familiar "dotted line" reporting structure and are able to respond to a dynamic external environment and remove barriers to cooperation. Some transplant programs have incorporated elements of both the functional and matrix reporting relationships (Figure 2.1). For example, some team members, such as pharmacists, social workers, and dieticians, may have a dotted line reporting relationship to those department heads in their

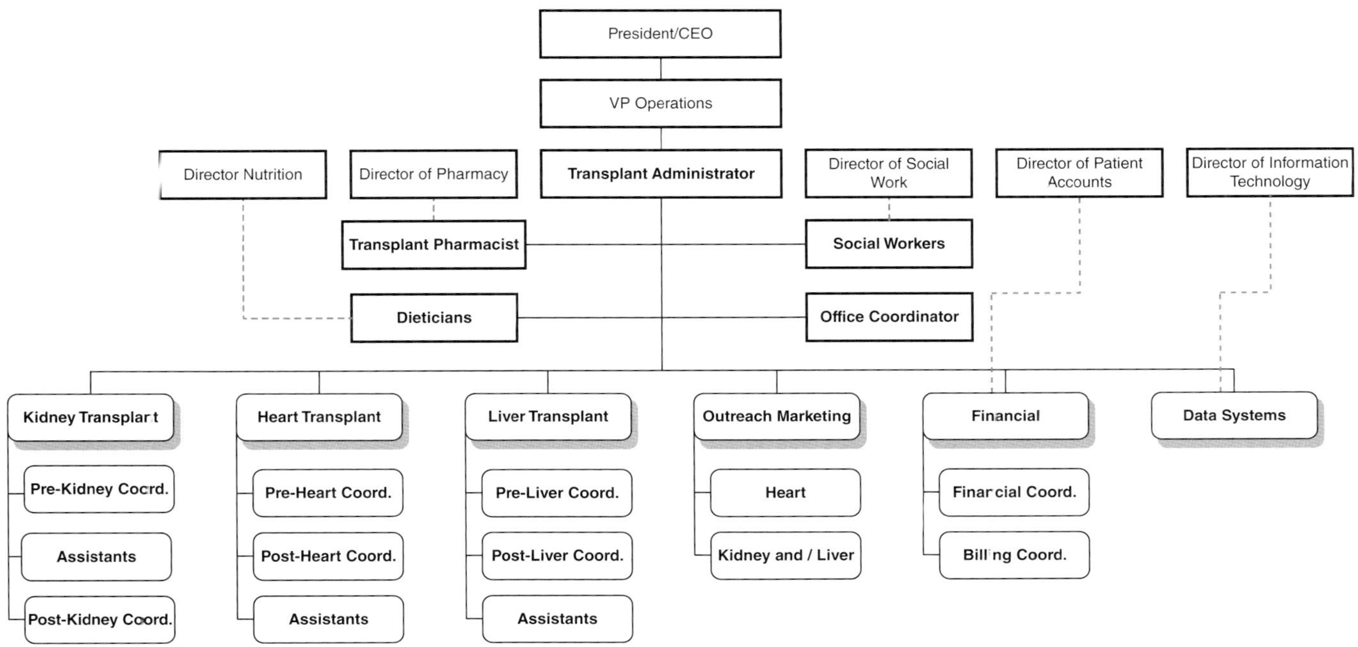

Figure 2.1 Matrix organization.

specialty. This dual accountability allows for training and networking in their profession. On the flip side, these same staff may have a dotted line reporting to the transplant administrator and direct reporting to each specialty head. This arrangement usually is not favorable since it may result in a "tug of war" for such resources and it introduces complexity in managing staff performance.

Advantages of a matrix structure:

- Improved ability to gain access to resources across the old functional silos.
- Better coordination on shared technologies across the organization (such as IT).
- Faster decentralized decisions.
- Multiskilled staff development.
- Better interfunctional cooperation.
- Better serves the needs of customers or patients.
- Supports a multidisciplinary team.

Disadvantages of a matrix structure:

- Power struggles between managers.
- Weak accountability.
- Requires more meetings and face-to-face interactions [2].

Service line structure

The service or product line organizational model emerged in the 1980s in response to a changing healthcare environment of managed care and increasing competition. This model integrates several hospital departments or functions into a service line whereby there is a consolidation of the financial, operational, clinical, marketing, and strategic functions. It can exist within the confines of an academic medical center but outside of the medical school departmental structure. It also can be found in the community hospital setting.

Increasing productivity, gaining economies of scale, and integrating patient care teams are some of the benefits of service lines [3]. It is the most common model for transplant programs since it is ideal in providing the infrastructure for a multidisciplinary team and the necessary control to ensure effective operations and growth. Typically, the transplant administrator reports to a chief operating officer, or vice president—in rare instances, he or she will report directly to the chief executive officer. Nonetheless, it is important for the administrator to "have the ear" of senior hospital leadership to secure necessary backing and financial resources. Figure 2.2 shows a typical service line structure. Questions that must be asked before moving to this structure are as follows:

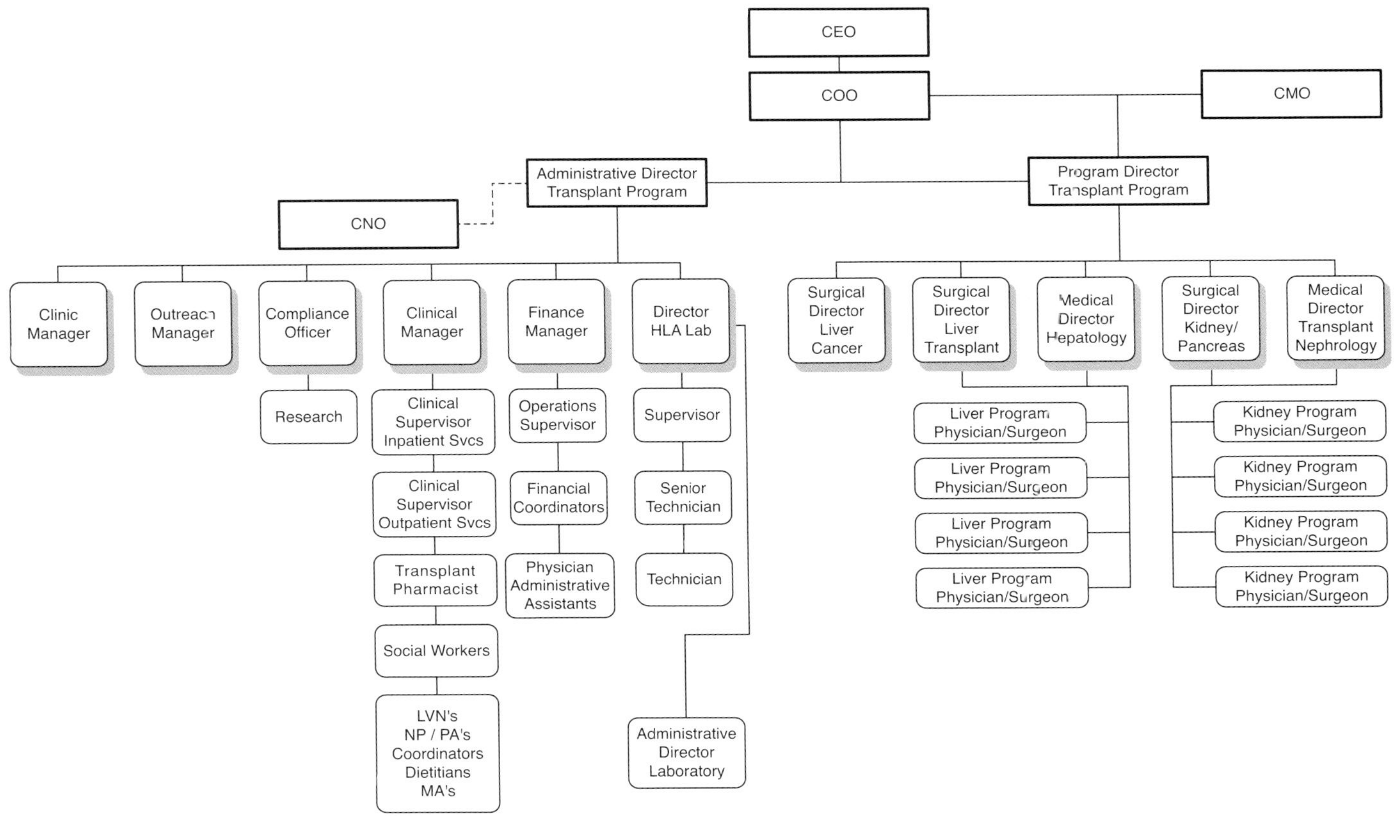

Figure 2.2 Service line organization.

- Is there the patient volume to support the development of this model?
- Is there a strong market for this service line?
- Will it be cost-effective?
- Are leaders from both the faculty and hospital committed to support this model?

Advantages of a service line structure:

- Provides patients with seamless, multidisciplinary care.
- Ease of contracting with managed care companies since services for the episode of care may be packaged.
- Competitive differentiation.
- Team has focus and develops a common culture.
- Ensures better regulatory compliance across all organ groups.
- Provides better integration of hospital leadership and faculty.

Disadvantages of a service line structure:

- Competition among service lines may create fragmentation.
- Potential increase in administrative overhead [4].

Institutes

The Miami Transplant Institute, The Georgetown Transplant Institute, and The University Hospitals Transplant Institute are a few of the transplant programs across the United States, but are they really institutes from an organizational perspective? It depends on definition. A survey of 20 transplant programs across the United States found that some transplant program respondents believed there was no difference between a transplant center and a transplant institute while others believed that an institute was independent and autonomous [5]. Transplant institutes are really financial joint ventures: the hospital and participating academic departments or private physician groups pool their resources and share the profits and expenses. Transplant Institutes can also be stand-alone enterprises which may contract with multiple hospitals to provide transplant care. In either case, they are few in number and difficult to form. In 2006, The Cleveland Clinic set on a course to form stand-alone institutes which are detailed in the following case study. The Clinic's reorganization to the institute model highlights how this structure supports integrated, multidisciplinary care which focuses on the patient experience. The challenges of this structural change were many, including a shift in culture, reporting relationships, leadership, and financial accountabilities. Although transplant services at the Cleveland Clinic are not structured in an institute model (the program cuts across several institutes at the Clinic), the program has a common administrative structure which ties it together. The lessons learned from this case study are applicable to any specialty in healthcare, including transplant.

Case study: Cleveland Clinic and the formation of institutes

Cleveland Clinic is a nonprofit, multispecialty academic medical center that integrates clinical and hospital care with research and education. It is world renowned for its outstanding patient care and outcomes. In 2011, the health system had more than 42,000 employees and 2700 physicians and scientists [1]. In addition to its network of hospitals in northeast Ohio, it has facilities in six US states and in Canada, and it oversees a facility in Abu Dhabi, United Arab Emirates.

In 2006, Dr Delos Cosgrove, the Clinic's CEO, embarked on a mission to redefine care delivery and expand geographically by reorganizing the Clinic into institutes, moving away from the traditional academic departmental model. These institutes were structured around diseases and organ systems with the hope that this new structure would improve the patient experience and emphasize wellness and prevention. Medical and surgical subspecialties would be grouped together, under the direction of an institute leader with financial accountability for both revenue and expenses. Each institute leader would be a respected physician or surgeon who was a proponent of team culture with an outstanding management track record. Obviously, this redefinition of reporting caused a radical upheaval in physicians and other staff, with the experience being described as "mixing matter with anti-matter" [2]. Physician concerns about title and rank also surfaced since institutes were not comparable to departments in academic medical centers. With regard to financial performance, the Clinic also had to redefine the way costs were assigned—away from cost per procedure or hospital day and toward cost per episode of care. They also moved to a common chargemaster and priced those services that were highly differentiated at a higher level than those that could be provided at a community hospital. In conjunction with this new structure was the implementation of a system-wide information system (EPIC) so that information could flow throughout the system and would appear seamless to patients.

By 2008, the reorganization and restructuring was completed and the task of measuring results began. The definition of success was going to be measured by patient experience, patient outcomes, and financial performance. As of 2011, results were impressive—outcomes, patient satisfaction, and market share had increased with financial performance, measured as operating income, increased by approximately $305 million [3].

References

1 Cleveland Clinic website. http://my.clevelandclinic.org/about-cleveland-clinic/overview/who-we-are/facts-figures.aspx
2 Porter M, Teisberg E. *The Cleveland Clinic: Growth Strategy 2008*. Boston, MA: Harvard Business School Publishing;2009.
3 Cleveland Clinic in Strong Financial Health–CEO, President Delos M. "Toby" Cosgrove, M.D., Delivers Annual "State of the Clinic" Address, *PR Newswire*, 2012.

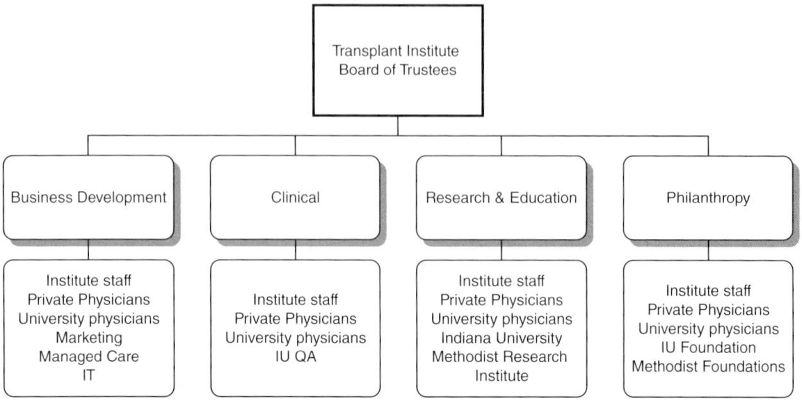

Figure 2.3 Indiana University Transplant Institute structure.
Source: Indiana University Transplant Institute © Indiana University Transplant Institute, with permission.

Indiana University (IU) Health Transplant Institute (formerly Clarian) in Indianapolis, Indiana, has been one of the few transplant programs that have actually formed a transplant institute model. This has been achieved by integrating existing resources along with private practice physicians into a free-standing entity. Figure 2.3 shows how the IU Transplant Institute is structured and the resources assigned to each subunit [6]. In IU's model, the physicians and hospital have clearly defined and understood the roles and responsibilities which are outlined contractually in physician service agreements. Physicians must be a part of managing the continuum of care which includes regulatory compliance, quality outcomes, cost management, and developing and adhering to standardized clinical protocols. In addition, physicians must participate in marketing, outreach, payor relations, research, and education and achieve certain predefined patient and referring physician satisfaction goals. In turn, the hospital also has the commitment to support capital projects and operating budget and provide support in the areas of marketing, information technology, human resources, and quality.

Advantages of an institute structure:

- It enhances the overall patient experience with integrated, multidisciplinary care.
- Control of transplant enterprise is in the hands of transplant leaders.
- Team culture is developed at its highest level.
- Responsibility and accountability lie within the institute.
- Well-understood financial contribution by the transplant enterprise.
- Ease of contracting with managed care organizations, i.e. global contracting.

Disadvantages of an institute structure:

- Politically challenging.
- Creates a shift in culture which is difficult to manage.
- Requires a large volume transplant enterprise to justify a stand-alone entity.
- Physician time spent on non-patient care activities related to the business.

No matter what the organizational structure may be, it is imperative that the hospital provides institutional commitment to the program. One of the most common reasons for transplant program turnover and regulatory difficulties is the lack of this key ingredient. It is incumbent upon transplant leadership to demonstrate to hospital senior leaders the value of the transplant program. This would include a strong business case highlighting the financial, clinical, and promotional aspects of having a program.

Conversely, hospital senior leaders must commit to make the transplant program a strategic priority, which will enable the program to sustain clinically sound operations, pursue innovation, and grow.

References

1 Daft, RL. *Organizational Theory and Design*. Mason, Ohio: Thomson South-Western; 2007:103.
2 Daft, RL. *Organizational Theory and Design*. Mason, Ohio: Thomson South-Western; 2007:111.
3 Turpinseed D, Lund DP, Sollenberger D. Product line development: a Strategy for clinical success in academic centers. *Ann Surg*. 246(4):585–592.
4 Daft RL. *Organizational Theory and Design*. Mason, Ohio: Thomson South-Western; 2007:105.
5 Abouljoud M, Klintmalm G, Whitehouse S. Transplant organizational structures: viewpoints from established centers. *Am J Transplant*. 12(10):2623–2629.
6 Institutional Vision and Commitment. (2011). Presentation at the transplant growth and management collaborative. retrieved from healthcare communities website: http://www.healthcarecommunities.org/SearchResults/ViewDocument.aspx?EntryId=49680. Accessed October 6, 2013.

CHAPTER 3
Human Resources

Lisa Norris
Transplant Leadership Institute LLC, San Antonio, TX, USA

Maintaining a healthy "exchange relationship," whereby income, recognition, and rewarding activities are exchanged for the work an employee performs is a key component of any business [1]. This relationship and its stability are vital not only for the overall organization, but also for a transplant program, to provide and sustain continued operations. Surgeons and physicians form the core of the transplant team with a multidisciplinary staff comprised of nurses, social workers, financial coordinators, pharmacists, administrative staff, and others, many of whom have highly specialized skills. Transplant staff serve as the gatekeepers and escorts of patients in the entire continuum of evaluation, transplant, and after-care; thus, it is critical for hospitals to provide a stable and satisfying work environment governed by policies that facilitate the recruitment and retention of talented, compassionate team members.

Much has been written on the topic of human resource management; however, transplant programs have unique requirements. The goal of this chapter was to guide readers through the issues and challenges of properly staffing a transplant program, successfully managing transplant personnel and creating a work environment that fosters the development and retention of dedicated team members.

Workforce planning

Planning for staffing needs of a transplant program is one of the many important challenges facing transplant leaders today. The demand for healthcare workers is ever increasing as our population grows and ages. Growth in the demand for nurses has already been felt in all areas of the United States and appears to be sustained due to the aging of the workforce. In 2012, the average age of a registered nurse (RN) is expected to be 44.7 years, with RNs in their 50's representing the largest group [2]. The average age of a transplant administrator is 49.3 years [3]. This aging

---

Transplant Administration, First Edition. Edited by Lisa Norris.

Companion website: www.wiley.com/go/norris/transplantadmin

phenomenon will greatly influence programs as to their hiring decisions and how they plan for their future workforce. Succession planning and identifying talented up-and-comers will become increasingly important for leadership.

The following are key reasons to engage in workforce planning:

- Assists in identifying surpluses and shortages in the workforce.
- Provides managers with tools to address changes in program direction that impacts that type of work being performed.
- Assists managers in creating a high-quality workforce capable of continually growing and changing.
- Helps in determining retirement projections and succession planning.
- Assists managers in identifying partnering, outsourcing, streamlining, and reorganizing opportunities.

Collection of data is the first step in workforce planning. The key data that should be collected are the following:

- Budget
- Changes in regulatory environment
- Benchmarking data
- Trends in the labor market
- New technology
- Trends in the competitive environment
- Market assessment
- Skills and skill mix
- Turnover rate
- Program coverage
- Patient-to-staff ratios

It is worth noting that this data has already led to changes in many transplant programs. Consider the labor force trend of a shortage of RNs and budgetary restraints, which has compelled most transplant programs to consider the role of a transplant assistant. Another example is the new Center for Medicare and Medicaid Services (CMS) regulatory requirements that have led to the addition of a new role of regulatory or compliance manager.

There is a balance between safe and effective care and the cost of care delivery. Budget constraints mandate that a sound business plan be developed for requesting additional personnel. Modifications and additions to staffing levels need to demonstrate an improvement in quality of care and return on investment. Most transplant programs focus on staff benchmarking data that are available on the UNOS Transplant Administrators website if the program has submitted their staffing data to UNOS for that year [4]. The program's data can then be compared against a number of factors: adult or pediatric, transplant volume, organ type, and UNOS region. Another method that can be used to determine appropriate staffing is the use of patient-to-staff ratios. The Transplant Leadership Institute recommended patient-to-staff ratio is roughly 165 patients to 1 coordinator based on our examination of many transplant programs over the years.

However, a word of caution is in order when using this benchmarking data. There is a tendency to assume that a program is over-staffed when staffing data are higher than the benchmarks or that the staff productivity is low. This may be the case; however, each program is unique. Therefore, a number of additional questions should be asked in order to right size the staff:

- Is the program pediatric or adult? Pediatric programs require a smaller staff-to-patient ratio to give more personalized care.
- Outreach clinics—do staff need to travel to do outreach in addition to their regular work?
- Does the program have an electronic medical record (EMR) or does it utilize paper charts? Paper charts require more staff to handle paper and organize records.
- Are the transplant coordinators staffing the clinics in addition to their workup or follow-up of patients? Clinic coverage will require more staff.
- Is the size of the waitlist large in comparison to the volume of transplants? The pretransplant workload is directly related to the number of patients being re-evaluated on an annual basis in addition to coordination of the evaluation of new patients.
- Do staff cover the continuum of care or do they specialize in one area? Coordinators in small transplant programs usually cover the continuum of care. As the volume increases, specializing becomes more efficient.
- Are patients followed post-transplant by the transplant program or referring physicians? Programs that have the responsibility of following patients indefinitely will require more staff.
- What is the experience level of staff? Those who are new to transplant will take longer to complete tasks.
- What type of nursing staff is required—nurse practitioners (NPs), RNs, or licensed practical nurses (LPN)? NPs are typically involved in post-transplant care, but are also employed in-patient in lieu of residents [5].
- How productive is the staff? Are there barriers to efficiently performing the work?

The last question regarding staff productivity should be examined in more depth. This is where there is the most opportunity to improve operations and budget. Focus on the most probable areas where inefficiency and waste occur: poor work layout, lack of technology, unclear work procedures and policies, and poor training. Further discussion of process improvement can be found in Chapter 8. An audit of transplant operations would be advised before hiring additional personnel.

Finally, it is sometimes necessary to create positions when there is a gap between the skills of current staff and the competencies that are needed by the program. At this point, a job description should be developed. Lists of duties of the various roles within a transplant program are found in Appendix 1, which will help in crafting a job description. Finally, if none of the existing staff possesses the necessary competencies or if training is not an option, recruitment for an external candidate should begin.

Recruitment and selection

In today's tough economic climate, it is difficult to find and attract top transplant talent. Highly qualified individuals at all levels are reluctant to leave secure jobs for an uncertain future in a different organization. In addition, relocation is also onerous and costly. Given the number of transplant programs in the United States, the pool of highly knowledgeable and experienced candidates is small. So, how does one begin? Several questions should be asked prior to the formal recruitment process:

- Should the program promote from within?
- Should the program find applicants who are less than fully qualified and provide additional training?
- Should the program consider agency, flexible staff, or outsourcing [6]?

The recruitment strategy selected depends on a realistic assessment of the availability of qualified internal talent, the requirements of the position, and the attractiveness of the transplant team and overall organization to qualified external applicants. Organizational attractiveness is influenced by geographic location, title, compensation, benefits, promotional opportunities, scope of responsibility, job security, and the values of the organization.

The recruitment process usually begins with a partnership between the human resource department of the organization and the transplant program. A position description is selected from an existing description or created for a new position. The importance of a clear, comprehensive, and accurate job description cannot be overstated: it provides a description of the desired attributes and the boundaries of the position responsibilities (see Appendix 1). A posting for the position is then crafted from the job description, and the posting is placed on the organization's website or job board. Candidates may also be sourced from employee referrals, networking in professional organizations, or recruiters. Identifying passive candidates or those not actively looking for employment is particularly important in increasing the candidate pool of qualified individuals with proven successful track records.

The number of qualified applicants received will be few in number as previously discussed. Although everyone would like to hire a superstar, an adjustment of expectations regarding current experience, job scope, and education may need to occur in order to uncover applicants who have transplant-related experience. Filling the position internally may also be an option if there are no external qualified candidates and may have several advantages: (i) it is less costly and time consuming, (ii) it indicates that the program is dedicated to develop talent from within, and (iii) the candidate is a known entity.

Once a pool of qualified candidates has been identified, the process of selection begins. Each candidate's experience and education is evaluated against the job specifications in the job description.

The most qualified candidates then progress to the interview process. At this point, the interview process can be broken down into three separate processes: candidate evaluation, selling the program to the candidate, and last, reaching interviewer consensus. Be aware that if there is too much emphasis on evaluation, the candidate may feel judged, which dampens enthusiasm for the position; too much selling may make the candidate feel like the program is desperate; and too much focus on consensus will prolong the process and top candidates might accept positions elsewhere [7].

Although this chapter will not delve into the myriad of interview techniques, the recognition of candidate "fit" is most critical in the selection process and the eventual developing of a satisfying work relationship between the organization and the employee. References should be asked about the candidate's style and workplace preferences, and they should be assessed against the current corporate culture. After the hire, particularly for administrators, assign a mentor to help them navigate the organization's political structure and unspoken norms and expectations.

Compensation

Individuals are motivated to work for many reasons—research on this topic has found that several factors are essential to job satisfaction: interest in the work, competent supervision, job environment, and, of course, compensation. Human resource professionals assert that money is not the prime motivating factor; however, it is usually near the top of the list especially in a small specialized field such as transplantation. A good compensation policy typically includes the following goals:

- Rewards performance
- Considers internal equity within the organization
- Ensures local market competitiveness
- Aligns performance with organizational goals
- Attracts and retains employees
- Maintains labor costs within the organizational budget [8]

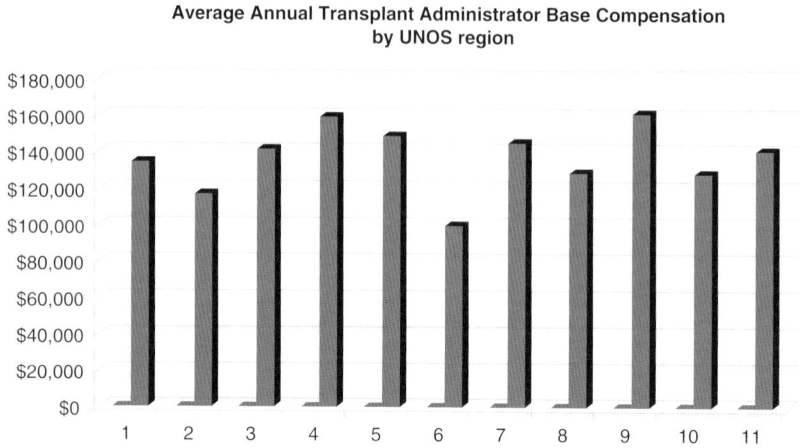

Figure 3.1 Average annual transplant administrator compensation 2010.

A transplant program typically must compete nationally for a small pool of qualified candidates. This situation drives compensation up, and hence conflict inevitably arises between internal equity and the ability to hire. In addition, the human resource department conducts market surveys to determine salary in the local market—the results of these surveys usually never include transplant professionals. In the past, transplant administrators have relied on word of mouth and calling other transplant programs to determine pay. Be aware that this gathering of salary information could constitute a potential violation of the Sherman Antitrust Act under salary fixing. The only way to limit exposure and potential liability is to use salary data from a third party.

It is important that the transplant director of the program have data to support the salaries of the various staff within the program. Most transplant staff professional organizations provided compensation surveys in the past, but have not updated them and are now unavailable. The only current compensation survey for transplant staff is for social workers which can be found at www.transplantsocialworker.org. Transplant administrator base compensation data have been collected by Transplant Leadership Institute (TLI) over the past 2 years and is shown in Figure 3.1. Approximately 48% of the administrators from the TLI data are eligible for a bonus, which is based on their respective organization's formula for meeting certain performance measures. The potential for these bonuses can be up to 20% of annual compensation.

Physician compensation and directorships

Most surgeons and physicians are compensated based on relative value units (RVUs), which is the methodology used by the Centers of Medicare

Table 3.1 Possible performance metrics for transplant surgeon/physician compensation

1	Decrease time from initial referral to waitlist by (*X*%) for those patients who have received financial clearance.
2	Maintain less than (*X*%) of patients on the waiting list as inactive status.
3	Ensure 100% compliance with CMS Conditions of Participation related to informed consent of potential transplant recipients and potential living donors.
4	Maintain patient survival rates (1 month, 1 year, and 3 year) within the expected ranges as calculated by the SRTR methodology.
5	Maintain graft survival rates (1 month, 1 year, and 3 year) within the expected ranges as calculated by the SRTR methodology.
6	Maintain patient satisfaction above the 90th percentile.
7	Length of stay less than or equal to established benchmark.

and Medicaid in determining professional reimbursement for clinical activity. RVUs certainly reflect productivity, but do not take into account the many other responsibilities and accountabilities that a physician/surgeon may have for the program [9]. To achieve better alignment between compensation and outcomes, additional performance metrics may be used to determine compensation as seen in Table 3.1.

All certified transplant programs require that medical and surgical leaders are in place in order to fulfill patient care and administrative duties. Most transplant centers have a compensation arrangement for these services; either they are employees of the hospital, members of an affiliated practice plan, or are contracted community physicians. Compensation for this required oversight of the transplant program can be reimbursed via the hospital cost report as a direct expense (also see Chapter 6 for more explanation). However, Stark Law enters into the equation and mandates that this compensation be based on the fair market value of physician time and cannot be based on the volume or value of any actual or anticipated referrals by the physician or the physician group. Failure to do so may result in criminal and/or civil penalties. Determination of fair market value can be determined in a variety of ways; however, use of multiple data sources and methodologies will ensure that the analysis is comprehensive and defendable under scrutiny. A detailed explanation can be found in the Federal Register at 42CFR 415.7 and 65 FR 5459 [10].

Compensation data for transplant physicians are available from a number of sources—Medscape, Medical Group Management Association, and Association of American Medical Colleges to name a few [11–13]. Compensation data for transplant surgeons can be found through the American Society of Transplant Surgeons [14]. Two companies that can provide specific and detailed assessment of physician compensation for a particular organization in a particular geographic location are Navigant and Sullivan Cotter & Associates.

Once the issue of compensation has been determined, job descriptions and contracts for physicians must be developed. Any agreement should include a detailed description of the services to be performed and should also set forth in detail the qualifications of the specific physician to provide the medical director or clinical services. Follow-up is necessary to ensure that the services are actually performed. The physician should be required to submit regular time records documenting the services. More will be written about Medical Directorships in Chapter 6. Job descriptions are ideal in communicating the scope of the role and the expectations. A sample job description for a medical/surgical director is found in Appendix 2.

Turnover and retention

Healthcare organizations had an average turnover rate of 14.6% in 2010 [15]. High turnover affects the quality of patient care and has high financial implications; for example, the estimated average cost of a single bedside nurse leaving an organization has been estimated to be between $36,000 to $48,000 [16]. Many factors influence turnover and retention. According to the Maryland Statewide Commission on the Crisis in Nursing, the primary reasons for nurse turnover are: (i) few advancement opportunities; (ii) stress and burnout; (iii) unrealistic workloads; (iv) increased paperwork; and (v) perception of lack of respect and recognition [17]. These reasons may also hold true for the various members of the transplant team. So what strategies can transplant leaders employ to enhance staff retention?

- Consider job sharing and flexible schedules.
- Develop and publicize promotional opportunities within the program.
- Clearly communicate job expectations and performance.
- Reward and recognize superior performance—formally or informally, publically and privately.
- Adequately compensate on-call duties.
- Support career development by providing continuing education or encouraging participation in professional societies/conferences.
- Help staff deal with work-related stress.
- Develop teamwork through teambuilding activities and celebrations.
- Staff the team adequately and provide coverage for vacations and absences.
- Develop and train an in-house transplant RN flex pool to cover absences.
- Listen. Solicit feedback from staff on work-related issues.
- Minimize time on paperwork and non-patient care activities.

- Address underperformance in a timely manner in order to minimize impact on the staff as a whole.

It is also necessary to consider transplant administrator turnover since administrators, as well as physician leaders, are providing the direction and operational oversight of the program. Our TLI research indicates that transplant administrator tenure is an average of 4 years [3]. Managing the complexity surrounding the transplant program is extremely challenging as previously discussed. In addition, navigating the political environment is difficult with many competing agendas among the key stakeholders. Causes of administrator turnover can range from poor program survey results, to burnout, to falling from the taut tightrope between physician leaders and hospital administration. There are several key items that help ensure success and retention of a transplant administrator:

- Development of an oversight committee so that decisions relating to the program involve all stakeholders.
- Development of a management team who reports to the administrator. This may be supervisors, lead coordinators, and/or managers, but the key concept is that there is a leadership team in place and that the responsibility of the program does not solely lie with the administrator.
- Supportive physicians and hospital administration who understand the business aspects of transplantation. If there is a gap in understanding, it behooves the transplant administrator to educate these key individuals.
- Emotional intelligence and the ability to work with physicians. Influencing physicians centers around building trust, creating efficiency and improvement in patient care, removing barriers, and valuing their time [18].

Training and advancement

Once the best candidate has been hired, the process of on-boarding or orientation sets the candidate on the path to success. Most candidates go through an organizational orientation program; however, there are many different policies, practices, and peculiarities associated with transplant programs. Developing a transplant-specific orientation manual is very helpful to new staff members. Ensuring that all staff are properly trained is important to the program, and documentation of such is mandated by the CMS transplant Conditions of Participation. Each individual should have in his or her personnel file a competency checklist of all the required tasks and properly signed off by the preceptor along with the job description. Orientation checklists for transplant coordinators and social workers are found in Appendices 3, 4, 5, and 6. The orientation period for transplant nurses spans many months and is typically accomplished through one-on-one preceptorships. If the new staff member has a limited knowledge of transplantation, books and resources about the clinical aspects of transplantation and the organ allocation system are very valuable. A good resource for both the new and experienced transplant nurse is the International Transplant Nurses Society IQ Series DVDs, which cover 16 topics on transplant nursing.

A common nursing issue in transplant programs is a lack of promotional opportunity. A Clinical Ladder program offers professional nurses the opportunity for career development and advancement while maintaining a clinical focus on patient care. It has been implemented in many hospitals in the United States; however, it is less commonly put into practice in transplant centers.

A Clinical Ladder program is a voluntary program in which the nurse demonstrates expertise in the areas of clinical management, educational activities, and research. It can be structured in a number of ways that would best suit the center and the nurses on the team. Examples of activities that might be considered for clinical ladder promotion are

- serving on transplant or hospital committees;
- providing education to other healthcare providers;
- precepting other staff members;
- publishing articles or abstracts;
- obtaining continuing education credits;
- participating in quality improvement initiatives;
- evaluating and utilizing nursing research;
- achieving specialty certification.

The application for promotion involves documenting all completed activities and interviews with a Clinical Ladder review committee and competency in the clinical setting. Research has shown that clinical ladder programs have increased nurse satisfaction, improved retention, and provided a financial benefit due to decreased turnover [19].

References

1 Griffith JR, White K. *The Well-Managed Healthcare Organization*. Chicago: Health Administration Press; 2007:465.
2 Auerbach DI, Buerhaus PI, Stanger DO. Better late than never: Workforce supply implications of later entry into nursing. *Health Aff*. 2007;26(1):178–185.
3 Transplant Leadership Institute. 2011. Internal data.
4 United Network for Organ Sharing. http://www.unos.org/transplant administrators.
5 Hoy H, Alexander S, Payne J, Zavala E. The role of advanced practice nurses in transplant center staffing. *Prog Transplant*. 2011;21(4):294–298.

6 Fried BJ, Gates M. Recruitment, selection and retention. In: Fried BJ, Fottler MD, eds. *Human Resources in Healthcare*. 3rd ed. Chicago: Health Administration Press; 2008:198–199.
7 Fernandez-Araoz C, Groysberg B, Nohria N. 2009. The Definitive Guide to Recruiting in Good Times and Bad. Harvard Business Review, May, p. 1–10.
8 Smith HL, Fried BJ, et al. Compensation practices, planning and challenges. In: Fried BJ, Fottler MD, eds. *Human Resources in Healthcare*. 3rd ed. Chicago: Health Administration Press; 2008:284.
9 Abouljoud MS. Innovative approaches to compensating and incentivizing the transplant professional: the virtual RVU. Abstract BPS-2. ASTS Winter Symposium 2011.
10 Federal Register 42CFR 415.70: Limits on compensation for physician services in providers. Federal Register 65 FR 45459: Updates to Reasonable Compensation Equivalent (RCE) Limits (415.70).
11 Medscape physician compensation survey. Medscape physician compensation survey. 2013. http://www.medscape.com/sites/public/physician-comp/2013. Accessed October 1, 2013.
12 Medical Group Management Association. www.mgma.com. Accessed October 1, 2013.
13 AAMC. www.aamc.org. Accessed October 1, 2013.
14 American Society of Transplant Surgeons. http://asts.org/resources/knowledge-base/transplant-surgeon-compensation-survey. Accessed October 1, 2013.
15 U.S. Department of Health and Human Services. Health Resources and Services Administration. 2007. The HRSA transplant center growth and management collaborative best practices final report. p. 23.
16 NSI Nursing Solutions Inc. 2013. National Healthcare and RN Retention Report. 2013: http://www.nsinursingsolutions.com/Files/assets/library/retention-institute/NationalHealthcareRNRetentionReport2013.pdf. Accessed October 1, 2013.
17 Maryland Statewide Commission on the Crisis in Nursing. 2001. Nurses Workplace Issues, Patient Safety, and the Quality of Patient Care.
18 Bujak J. *Inside the Physician Mind*. Chicago: Health Administration Press; 2008:53–54.
19 Drenkard K, Swartwout E. Effectiveness of a clinical ladder program. *J Nurs Adm*. 2005;35(11):502–506.

CHAPTER 4
Clinical Services

Lisa Norris
Transplant Leadership Institute LLC, San Antonio, TX, USA

The clinical aspects of a transplant program range from pre-transplant evaluation to post-transplant patient management and all that it entails: testing, clinic visits, in-patient stay, medications, psychosocial evaluation, dietary needs, and the list goes on. Although this chapter will not delve into these clinical aspects, it is extremely important for those managing a transplant program to have a basic understanding of the science of transplantation, donor and patient selection, organ allocation, and in-patient and post-transplant patient management for each of the solid organs. This chapter covers the business aspects of managing the clinical side of transplantation and attempts to answer the following questions: (i) How can a transplant program create convenient access for patients? (ii) How can referrals be increased? (iii) How can patients be efficiently managed during the entire continuum of care? (iv) What are some of the best practices in decreasing cost?

Referral and access

Broadening the referral base and creating many avenues for access to transplant services should be one of the main goals of any transplant program. Apart from marketing efforts and managed care contractual arrangements to obtain referrals, most referrals come from specialty providers. Cultivating a good relationship with these specialists is very important and rests on the provision of the following:

- Specialty providers seek clinical judgment and advice from transplant physicians and surgeons in a timely manner. This establishes a strong collegial relationship that will result in a lasting referral stream.
- They expect easy transfer of critically ill patients to the transplant hospital, which should have adequate ICU and bed capacity.
- These providers want patient information on the status of evaluation, abnormal test results, timely listing, transplant status, and updates on post-transplant care.

Transplant Administration, First Edition. Edited by Lisa Norris.

Companion website: www.wiley.com/go/norris/transplantadmin

- Most providers want to see their patients return to their practice post-transplant for both clinical and financial reasons (kidney, in particular). Try to establish a close partnership with them.

Cleveland Clinic provides an excellent example of an organization that has put thought into cultivating the referring physician relationship and has created easy ways for referring physicians to obtain information and provide access. They have developed a transplant referral phone line, a referring physician center for service-related issues and information about the Clinic's specialists, a transfer phone line for hospital transfers, a critical care transport team, mobile ICU vehicles, online access to patient information, and online access to the latest outcomes data [1].

Another way to grow a referral base and to improve access is to establish satellite clinics in areas where there are no transplant programs nearby or the journey to the transplant center is burdensome and costly to the patient. Some patients simply cannot afford multiple trips to the transplant center for evaluation and testing. Developing an outreach program is an excellent way to grow the referral base and provides a tremendous service to patients in outlying areas. A recent study showed that referrals to a transplant program from two outlying geographic areas increased 80% and 270%, respectively, when a satellite clinic was initiated [2]. Indeed, many transplant programs have developed these clinics; however, there are hurdles to be overcome that are logistical, legal, and financial, which should be considered:

- Clinic space—space can be leased or some programs have established clinics in existing physician offices or hospital facilities. The latter arrangements must be carefully examined with anti-kickback laws in mind [3].
- Scheduling the team and impact on existing workload—getting the necessary team assembled for a satellite clinic is one obstacle; however, the biggest challenge is how to manage the existing work and the surge of new work that is brought back from the satellite clinic. One way to deal with the workload is to develop coordinator/assistant teams. While the nurse is conducting an outreach clinic, the assistant can carry forward some of the work. This will alleviate the burden and stress on transplant coordinators.
- Evaluation testing performed within the local community—testing from outside providers necessitates that a contract be in place with the transplant hospital since payment for all pretransplant testing is the responsibility of the transplant hospital. Also, tracking and receiving results from many different providers pose a challenge for transplant coordinators and the effect is additional workload. Last, but not least, any evaluation testing that is not performed in the transplant hospital is less

profitable for the program since internal cost is much less than for purchased services.

- Billing issues—all facility and professional fees for the pretransplant phase are billed to the transplant hospital. Facility fees can only be charged if the clinic space has been leased. All post-transplant care is billed to Medicare, Medicaid, or insurance.

Finally, access for the transplant program can be improved by establishing housing for overnight and extended stays. This housing may be family houses, hotels and/or motels with special rates, Ronald McDonald houses, apartments, or converted dormitories. No matter the housing option, it should be convenient and low cost in order for patients and their families to economically stay for evaluation and later during transplant peri- and postoperative care. Transplant programs who have established some type of low-cost housing alternatives are definitely at a competitive advantage—access is easier and managed care organizations also place a high value on the availability of housing for their members.

Pretransplant evaluation

The typical pretransplant process has been flowcharted as seen in Figure 4.1. The referral is made to the transplant coordinator. The transplant coordinator enters information into the transplant database, calls the patient to get demographic and health history, and sends a packet of information to the patient if the patient has no health conditions that rule out transplantation. The patient information is sent to the financial coordinator who obtains payor authorization and then enters the insurance information into the hospital billing system. The patient's medical records are requested and then the patient is scheduled for a clinic visit. Table 4.1 summarizes the staff members of a typical transplant clinic and their duties. During the clinic visit, the patient receives education about the transplant process—group educational sessions are the most efficient and effective. Next, the patient has an appointment with either a surgeon or a physician (or both), and their blood is drawn for serological and other tests. The patient is given orders for the remainder of the evaluation testing. It is the responsibility of the patient to make appointments with a variety of providers either at the transplant hospital or externally for these tests and communicate the progress to the transplant coordinator. If the patient requires external testing, the transplant coordinator is placed in a position of not knowing exactly where the patient is in the evaluation process and has to spend an inordinate amount of time tracking down test results. This entire pretransplant process could potentially take up to a year or more to complete. A study at Yale University School

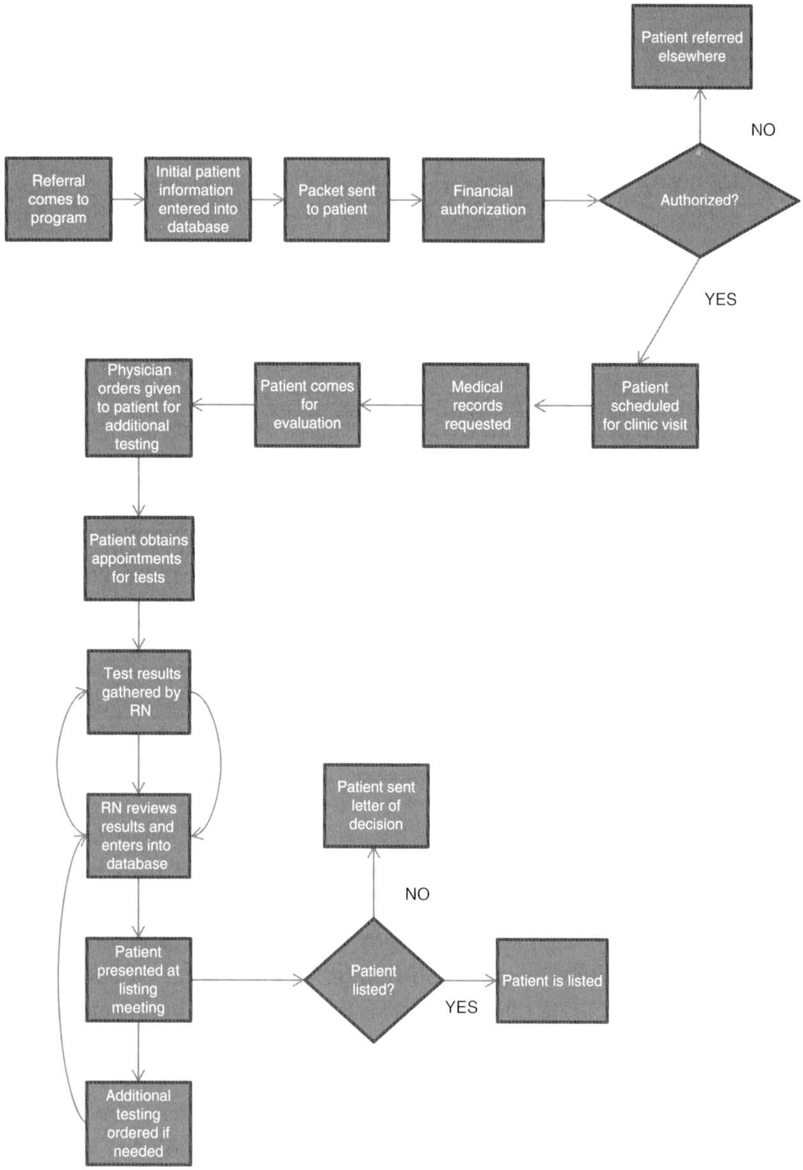

Figure 4.1 Pretransplant evaluation process for recipients.

of Medicine retrospectively evaluated 905 patients waiting for kidney transplant. Of the total number of patients, 378 patients were evaluated by the process discussed earlier and 578 patients were evaluated during a one-day process. The group undergoing a traditional evaluation had a median referral to listing time of 226 days, whereas the group undergoing a one-day evaluation had a median referral to listing time of 46 days [4]. Many transplant programs have realized that they must increase the throughput of patients in the pretransplant evaluation process by

Table 4.1 Staffing of transplant clinic

Role	Duties
Transplant Coordinator	• Perform patient education • Review medications with patients • Examine wounds and perform wound care as needed • Perform post-op observations • Admits to hospital • Assess patients • Assign clinic charges • Performs care coordination
Administrative Assistant or Scheduler	• Schedules patient for visit and/or future visits
Medical Assistant	• Rooms patient • Takes vital signs • Draws labs
Receptionist	• Greets and signs in patients • Answers phones • Ask patient about any insurance or demographic changes • Ensures waiting room is tidy

decreasing the time of referral to waitlisting in order to minimize dialysis exposure. This trend benefits patients in accumulating more time on the list (for kidneys) at least under the current allocation system and decreases the accumulation of comorbid conditions prior to transplant. So, how do programs accomplish a one-day evaluation?

The word that best describes it is "fast-tracking." Fast-tracking is a process whereby a patient is scheduled for all necessary consults and tests over several days to complete transplant evaluation. This is achieved by first having the patient attend educational sessions and meet with the financial coordinator. Once cleared financially for transplant, the patient is either admitted for testing or, in the case at Yale, admitted to their infusion center for testing. Next, the patient meets with the surgeon, the physician, social worker, and dietician to review all the results and determine if any additional testing is needed. The process for various patient types can be seen in Figure 4.2. Although this process improves patient throughput, is convenient for the patient, and may result in an increase in the volume of transplants, the in-patient stay is not reimbursed by Medicare or private payors. A careful review of the costs versus benefits would be necessary before initiating a fast-track process.

Waitlist management

Waitlist management is a hot topic particularly for kidney transplant programs with large waiting lists. It is not unheard of in the kidney transplant

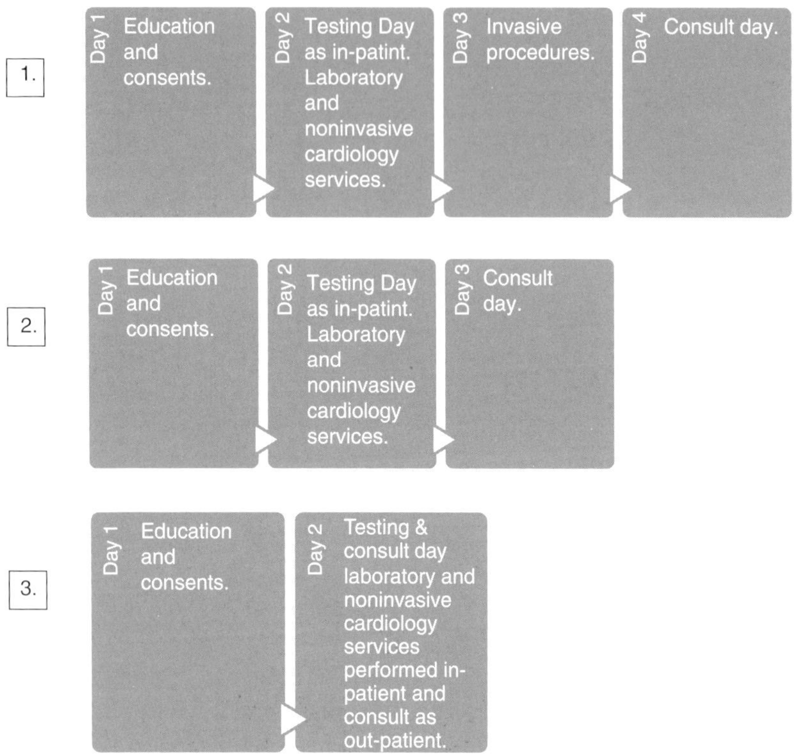

Figure 4.2 Fast-tracking evaluation process: (1) complex patient; (2) standard patient; (3) out of town patient.

community to have a top 10 list for each blood group in order to ensure that these patients near the top of the list are prepared. But, what about the remainder of patients who are waitlisted? Obviously, it is extremely time consuming to manage this population due to the prevalence of chronic diseases and the long waiting time on the list. Properly managing the waitlist will result in patients who are clinically ready for transplantation at the time an organ is available and will decrease mortality on the waitlist. Past studies found that waitlist management of patients was highly variable, with 18% of transplant centers doing no re-evaluation at all [5]. According to a recent study by Vanderbilt University, 80% of the 59 responding transplant programs re-evaluated their patients at transplant center predefined time intervals. In all cases, those programs with a dedicated waitlist coordinator showed a decrease in patient mortality while waiting compared to those who did not [6]. This waitlist management function can be performed internally by dedicated staff or outsourced to one of the firms who specialize in providing this service.

There are also several methods to reduce organ acquisition cost as it relates to waitlisted patients. First, since there are costs associated with listing and being maintained on the list, only list those patients who have no contraindications and delist those who, for health reasons, no longer qualify [7]. In addition, panel reactive antibody testing that used to be performed each month on each waitlisted patient can now be performed quarterly. This new standard in testing can save a program several hundreds of thousands of dollars per year, not to mention the staff time in managing results without any effect on organ offers [8]. The bottom line for the transplant administrator is that good waitlist management is necessary and cost-effective—that having resources to perform this task is one of the foundations for good clinical care.

Organ turn downs

The organ refusals for any transplant program should be reviewed monthly. The data can be found in the Report of Organs Offered and Transplanted (ROOT) on the UNet website. This report contains a list of the organ offers that were either transplanted or turned down for transplant that eventually were transplanted at another program, and it is updated on a monthly basis. Some of the data included on the report is:

- Was the offer accepted?
- Reason for refusal.
- Local or imported.
- Donor characteristics.
- Who eventually received the organ?
- Outcome and survival (graft functioning/failed, graft survival time).

Why is this important? This report can help the surgical team determine whether they are being too conservative or too liberal in accepting organ offers. It can also identify trends so that practices can be changed. Also, it may point out that team coverage is inadequate. Ultimately, if the program is refusing organs that are successfully being transplanted at another program, then volume, profitability, and good patient care are being affected.

In-patient

There are several keys to efficiently and effectively managing the transplant in-patient. Patients with shorter lengths of stay will have lower costs, which translates to higher margins on cases. Many issues that contribute to longer lengths of stay are inadequate understanding of patient education material, lack of timely discharge, insurance authorization issues, and lack of transportation, among others. Having an in-patient coordinator is the key to addressing these patient care issues and decreasing cost in the in-patient setting. This coordinator could be rotated among existing post-transplant coordinators or a dedicated position filled by either a transplant coordinator or a nurse practitioner. A nurse practitioner has more versatility and can function within a broader scope in that they typically have prescribing authority and the ability to admit and discharge [9]. Many times, in an academic medical center, in-patient nurse practitioners serve as surrogates to residents and provide the education and continuity that is needed on the in-patient unit. Large transplant programs also utilize the services of a case manager in addition to an in-patient coordinator to further facilitate discharge.

Review and revision of in-patient clinical pathways is also important in minimizing expenses to increase margins in this era of continuing reductions in reimbursement from public and commercial payors. A team should be assembled with physicians and staff to map out the process from admission to discharge in order to determine where the opportunities are to reduce cost. First, tackling the low hanging fruit would be recommended. Length of stay (LOS) is the single best area to concentrate efforts since it has the most impact on overall in-patient cost. Examination of practice patterns regarding admission is advisable—look at the practice of admitting living donors and recipients the day before surgery. Consider delays surrounding discharge and remove any obstacles. It is advisable to routinely track the LOS on a quarterly basis and present the findings to the QAPI committee. Other tactics to manage cost should include review of the utilization of other services. It is key to involve physicians and surgeons in the discussion of this utilization data and obtain their buy-in to practice changes. Some other services that could be looked at are:

- evaluating the frequency of intravenous antibiotic therapy;
- evaluating induction therapies;
- laboratory test and imaging frequency.

Post-transplant

Patients who undergo transplantation usually are followed postoperatively at the transplant center as long as they live. It is understandable that the transplant team would want to ensure that the patients are closely monitored in order to maintain good outcomes and often times becomes the primary care provider for the transplant patient. This creates three dilemmas: As the program transplants more and more transplant patients, the number of post-transplant patients who are followed rapidly expands. This situation requires adding more post-transplant staff to the program even though revenue and profit may not be favorable. Second, post-transplant care is not reimbursable via the cost report but by Medicare, Medicaid, and private insurers. Typically, revenue from post-transplant clinic operations does not cover the expense of clinic operations in addition to the post-transplant care team (see discussion in Chapter 6). Lastly, the complexity of these patients and necessity for timely response can force transplant coordinators to operate outside their scope of practice. So what can be done to manage this population given these issues? One good solution to the first two dilemmas is to transition most of the patients to their referring physician for follow-up and general health maintenance. The readiness and level of comfort of the referring physician in caring for the post-transplant patient may vary depending on the organ transplanted. However, many programs have been creative in supporting referring physicians by offering educational seminars, and some have in fact developed a "transplant university." This "university" concept is built around shadowing the program's transplant physicians for a week in order to develop proficiency in managing immunosuppression and recognizing infection, and acute and chronic rejection.

Many coordinators have shared that they have been placed in situations where they operate outside of their scope of practice. This creates an uncomfortable situation for any nurse since potentially their nursing license may be at stake. The post-transplant arena poses the most risk for this type of situation. Transplant coordinators typically work under standing orders or obtain a verbal or written order from the physician [8]. In practicality, this is difficult to do with hundreds of patients to manage. In theory, all patient results must be reviewed by a physician or provider; unfortunately this does not always occur. A solution for transplant centers is to employ nurse practitioners as post-transplant coordinators since they function under the direction of a physician, but can practice independently. The duties of a nurse practitioner typically are monitoring of immunosuppression and taper per protocol, see patients in clinic, and follow-up with patients regarding other health issues [10, 11].

Finally, documentation of the post-transplant clinic visit by nurses must be comprehensive and support services rendered in order for facility fees to be billed to Medicare patients. The Center for Medicare and Medicaid Services (CMS) has mandated that hospitals must have a documented process for determining facility fee levels; however, they have not stipulated a specific process. Typically, facility fees are billed using Evaluation and Management codes from Current Procedural Terminology manual along with the quantity of nursing time used for delivering care. Properly documenting clinic visits will result in the maximum reimbursement for services. In addition, as clinic volume increases, the increase in facility fees can provide the necessary justification for additional nursing staff. A guide for determining facility fees for a post-transplant clinic is given in Table 4.2.

Table 4.2 Ambulatory clinic visit charge sheet

Clinic Visit CHARGES			**Circle the appropriate Level Charge**
Level 1	99201 new	99211 established	***new** = a patient not seen within the last three years as inpatient or outpatient
Level 2	99202 new	99212 established	
Level 3	99203 new	99213 established	***established** = a patient that has been registered as an inpatient or outpatient **in the last 3 years** at the facility
Level 4	99204 new	99214 established	
Level 5	99205 new	99215 established	

†**CLINIC Contributory Factors may increase visit assignment by one level and only one factor is required:** Contributory Factors include: non-verbal patient, patient age less than 8 years, need for two or more staff simultaneously to provide care, arrival by EMS or private ambulance, or discharge to anywhere other than home

Level 1	Level 2	Level 3		Level 4 - 99284	Level 5 - 99285
Weight check	Cleaning and dressing simple wounds	Administration of an single enema	Care coordination with outside agencies of less than 30 minutes	Care coordination with outside agencies >30 min	Multiple enemas
Blood Pressure Check		Irrigation of bag and/or dressing change of central lines, ostomy or other devices	Generalized disease-related teaching of 15-30 minutes	Removal of an established line, stent	Extensive Photo documentation of bodily injuries
Suture Removal		Crutch walk teaching	Application of "off the shelf" orthopedic supply device	suctioning of endotracheal or NG or oral gastric tubes	
Phlebotomy draw			Simple photo documentation required for the assessment of less than 5 photos	Tracheal suctioning via tracheostomy	Freq monitoring as evidence of 3 sets of V/S/ assessments integral to the patients condition or interventions.

Review of lab results with patient face to face	Administration of one oral or rectal or topical medication	Multiple oral, topical, rectal medications	Psychiatric coordination, consultation and precertification in an non-behavioral health setting	*Oxygen administration (includes conversion to hospital supplied with rate adjustments)	Assessment, crisis intervention and supervision on imminent behavior crisis threatening to harm self or others
Physician counseling of patient requiring use of exam room/facility	Behavioral Health data collection	Freq monitoring as evidence by 2 sets of V/S/ assessments integral to the patient's condition or interventions		Floor admission	ICU/OR Admit
	Assist with MD exams with supportive nursing documentation	Assist patient with 2 or more activities of daily life (eating, toiletry, dressing, etc)		Consult with social worker, dietician, and/or childlife	Tele/IMC Admit
				Specialized education by an internal certified educator	Transfer to the Emergency Department
RN Signature:			Patient Label		

References

1 Cleveland Clinic Transplantation Annual Report. 2010. p. 91.

2 Detwiler R, et al. Developing transplant outreach clinics: a collaborative marketing and clinical success story. Abstract presented at the Transplant Management Forum. 2012.

3 Program Integrity—Medicare and State Health Care Programs. Title 42, *Code of Federal Regulations*, Pt. 1001.952, 2011 ed. p. 735.

4 Formica RN, Barrantes F, Asch WS, et al. A one day centralized workup for kidney transplant recipient candidates: a quality improvement report. *Am J Kidney Dis*. 2012;60(2):288–294.

5 Zarifian A, O'Rourke M. Managing the kidney waiting list. *Prog Transplant*. 2006; 16(3):242–246.

6 Wu S, et al. Waitlist management in kidney transplant programs: a practical review. 2012. Abstract presented at the Transplant Management Forum.

7 Abecassis M. Organ acquisition cost centers Part II: reducing the burden of cost and inventory. *Am J Transplant*. 2006;6(12):2838.

8 Grote, T. HLA monitoring is an effective tool for transplant program cost reduction and improved waitlist management. 2012. Abstract presented at the Transplant Management Forum.

9 Tedesco J. Acute care nurse practitioners in transplantation. *Prog Transplant*. 2011; 21(4):279.

10 Tedesco J. Acute care nurse practitioners in transplantation. *Prog Transplant*. 2011;21(4):280.

11 Hoy H, Alexander S, Payne J, et al. The role of advanced nurse practice nurses in transplant center staffing. *Prog Transplant*. 2011;21(4):297.

CHAPTER 5
Regulatory and Compliance Issues

Marguerite Brown
Laurel Avenue, Menlo Park, CA, USA

The delivery of organ transplantation services has become one of the most highly regulated clinical activities within the hospital and outpatient setting. Noncompliance with agency requirements may result in serious consequences which can ultimately threaten the viability of the transplant program. A thorough understanding of the required elements to meet the regulatory requirements for each agency and a process dedicated to ensuring ongoing compliance is an essential capability for the transplant administrator. Although the administrator is often considered the primary team member held accountable for meeting agency requirements, the respective program physician leaders also play an integral role in promoting adherence to policies and documentation processes required for regulatory compliance. Due to the complexity and critical importance of regulatory compliance, many transplant centers have appointed dedicated personnel in the role of a Quality and Regulatory Manager to ensure adequate attention is devoted to this area. Individuals charged with these responsibilities must be provided with the support and necessary resources to maintain knowledge of changing regulations and implement new processes for auditing compliance. Transplant centers must provide the highest quality clinical care to patients receiving transplant services and for those individuals who serve as living donors.

There are many regulatory agencies with oversight of organ transplantation, and they include the Organ Procurement and Transplantation Network (OPTN)/United Network for Organ Sharing (UNOS), Centers for Medicare and Medicaid Services (CMS), Department of Health and Human Services (DHHS), the End-Stage Renal Disease Network (ESRD), State Department of Health and Human Services (SDHHS), The Joint Commission (TJC), and the Office of the Inspector General (OIG).

Beginning in 2007, there has been a focused effort on the part of both the OPTN/UNOS and CMS to hold transplant programs accountable for meeting all of the respective requirements for these agencies. The ultimate

Transplant Administration, First Edition. Edited by Lisa Norris.

Companion website: www.wiley.com/go/norris/transplantadmin

goal for these actions has been to improve the clinical outcomes and overall safety aspects and quality of transplantation services.

CMS regulations

The federal government began regulating kidney transplantation in 1976 under the Code of Federal Regulation (CFR). Coverage decisions were made by CMS in regard to heart transplants in 1987, liver transplants in 1991, lung transplants in 1995, and intestine transplants in 2001. On March 30, 2007, CMS published the final regulations for transplant programs in the Federal Register, and they became effective 90 days later on June 28, 2007. The document had 440 pages and contained the new regulations and additional information, which defined the *Medicare Conditions of Participation for transplant hospitals* (CoPs) 42 CFR Part 482. As of April, 2012, there were 239 transplant hospitals in the United States which housed 787 different Medicare certified programs [1]. Hospitals must comply with the extensive regulations in order to secure or maintain certification to provide transplant services for patients with Medicare funding. In order for a new program to apply to be approved by Medicare, they must submit a request to CMS Central Office. There is no application form. A list of the information that a provider must submit with their application for approval is posted on the CMS Survey and Certification website http://www.cms.gov/Medicare/Provider-Enrollment-and-Certification/CertificationandComplianc/Downloads/Combinedappinfo.pdf.

Assistance in meeting the regulations is provided by CMS to survey agencies and contractors through a set of interpretive guidelines. The interpretive guidelines contain authoritative interpretations, clarifications of the regulatory requirements, and examples to support the regulatory text. They are available at http://www.cms.gov/Medicare/Provider-Enrollment-and-Certification/SurveyCertificationGenInfo/downloads/SCLetter08-25.pdf. The guidelines are an aide and do not replace or supersede the law or regulation, and therefore cannot be used as the documentation basis for a citation. The guidelines are critical for the transplant facility to use in order to ensure their policies, consents, and transplant process documentation contain the essential elements that surveyors need to attest as sufficient to meet the regulation when they conduct their audit.

In addition to meeting various process requirements, transplant programs must maintain appropriate communication with CMS. Programs are required to notify the agency within 7 days of any major changes to the program that could affect its compliance with Medicare's CoP under 42 CFR 482.74. These areas include changes in key staff members, a decrease

Table 5.1 Content for the Transplant Program Quarterly Report (TPQR) provided by OPTN to CMS

- Contact information for representatives of the hospital and transplant program;
- Survey and certification information including the survey priority, status, and approval or re-approval due date (if applicable);
- Affiliations including membership with the OPTN, and an agreement with an organ procurement organization;
- Key personnel of the transplant program (i.e., the primary transplant surgeon and transplant physician);
- Program data including data submission, the number of transplant performed, and the program's outcomes; and
- Notifications of program changes and inactivity.

in the number of transplants performed, a decrease in the program's survival rates, or the termination of an agreement between the hospital and the organ procurement organization (OPO) and inactivation of the transplant program.

The certification regulations consist of two types of requirements. These are categorized as "process" requirements and requirements related to outcomes, clinical experience (volume), and data submission rates. Clinical outcome data are published biannually (January and July) by the Scientific Registry of Transplant Recipients (SRTR.org) and will be further discussed in Chapter 9. The OPTN provides information for volume and data submission rates. Volume metrics and data submission requirements are acquired without onsite visits and are contained within the Transplant Center Quarterly Report (TPQR) which is provided to surveyors through the CMS Central Office. The TPQR uses the most recent Program-Specific Report from the SRTR and will note whether the 1-year post-transplant patient and graft survival is lower than expected and (i) the one-sided p-value is less than 0.05; (ii) the number of observed events minus the expected events is greater than 3; and (iii) the number of observed events divided by the number of expected events is greater than 1.5.

All content for the TPQR is noted in Table 5.1. Surveyors will confirm that the content for the TPQR can be validated as accurate during the onsite survey. Along with other requirements, they will confirm that any changes in key personnel with regard to the UNOS primary surgeon and physician were appropriately relayed and updated within the timeframe required by CMS.

CMS surveys

Survey process

Routine onsite re-certification surveys are conducted approximately every 3 years. Surveys can also occur at any time when a specific complaint

Table 5.2 List of states surveyed by state agency or national contractors

National contractors	State survey agencies	
Alabama	Arizona	Tennessee
Arkansas	California	Texas
Colorado	Florida	Virginia
Connecticut	Georgia	Washington
Delaware	Illinois	
Hawaii	Indiana	
Louisiana	Iowa	
Maine	Kansas	
Mississippi	Kentucky	
Nebraska	Maryland	
Nevada	Massachusetts	
New Hampshire	Michigan	
New Mexico	Minnesota	
Oregon	Missouri	
Rhode Island	New Jersey	
South Carolina	New York	
Utah	North Carolina	
Vermont	North Dakota	
West Virginia	Ohio	
Wisconsin	Oklahoma	
	Pennsylvania	
	South Dakota	

made by a patient or other entity appears to be a "credible allegation" of a condition-level deficiency. Individual states will have surveys conducted by a state agency or through a federal contractor (Healthcare Management Solutions). Table 5.2 displays the states surveyed by state agencies and those surveyed by the federal contractor. One to two surveyors will generally be assigned to each type of organ transplant program and, depending on the number of programs surveyed, will spend three to six working days at the facility. The visit to the transplant hospital is made with no prior notification; therefore, centers need to maintain a "survey ready" status at all times.

Upon entry to the facility, surveyors will go to the hospital's administrative offices and announce their arrival and purpose. They will conduct an "Opening Conference," which provides an overview of their process and projected date and time for an "Exit Conference." Senior hospital administrators and physician leaders should attend both sessions along with members of the transplant team such as nurse coordinators, social workers, and other support personnel. A list of 34 items divided into eight categories will be requested by the surveyors. These items are listed in

Table 5.3. Some of the requested materials include lists of candidates, recipients, living donors, organ recoveries, and organ offers. Also reviewed are specific program policies, a list of personnel and their titles, and information regarding quality assessment and process improvement (QAPI) activities.

The number of patient charts chosen for auditing will be determined based on a program volume metric. Depending on the size of the waiting list or the number of transplants performed per year, three to eight charts will be reviewed. Transplant personnel will be interviewed regarding their role, patients will be interviewed regarding their experience, and consents and other documents will be reviewed to assure language content is in compliance with the CMS regulations. Surveyors should be provided a secure place to work and have access to photocopy and fax machines as well as several computers in order to access the electronic medical records (EMRs). If records dating back to the 3-year period under review are in paper form, these charts must also be secured and on-site for the survey. Generally, transplant nurse coordinators for the respective transplant programs will assist the surveyors in the review of patient records. The individuals chosen for this task must be adept at navigating the EMR or paper charts in order to locate the documentation requested in a timely manner.

After surveyors complete their review, an "Exit Conference" will be held and a verbal report of the surveyors' findings is provided to those in attendance. Information is shared regarding any deficiencies found onsite as well as any within the TPQR. Examples are given as to specifically how the program was found noncompliant with a condition-level deficiency or with standards necessary to meet a condition of participation (CoP). The program is given the opportunity to rebut the findings by presenting additional information. It is always important to try and find the type of documentation that can meet the surveyor's request before they leave the facility in order to avoid a citation. During the verbal report, surveyors will explain that all findings are preliminary and subject to administrative review by CMS Central Office. A final written report will be sent to the hospital which delineates all of the deficiencies. The timeline to receive this report is generally within 10 business days, but there can be delays.

Final report and response

The outcome for a survey is officially communicated through a letter sent to the hospital CEO or chief regulatory representative. The letter will state the findings of the survey and categorize the deficiencies as falling into two categories—condition level or standard level. The details for the citations are provided through a form referred to as CMS-2567. A condition-level citation is the most serious deficiency and indicates that the center has failed to meet a specific required CoP to provide transplant services. Often,

Table 5.3 List of items requested by CMS surveyors at start of onsite visit

List of transplant candidates, recipients, and living donors

1 The transplant program's complete current active waiting list including the following information: name, address, country of primary residence, resident alien or non-resident alien status, race and gender, and number of individuals on the waiting list (not status 7 patients);
2 List and number of patients removed from the waiting list including the reason for the removal within the past 12 months (removed due to death or transplant);
3 List and number of all persons removed from the waiting list over the past 12 months for reasons other than death or transplant;
4 List and number of persons evaluated for transplant that were not placed on the waiting list within the last 12 months; do not include persons that are currently in the evaluation process;
5 List and number of the transplants performed including name, organ(s) transplanted, address, country of primary residence, resident alien status or non-resident alien status, race and gender, and date of transplant within the past 3 years;
6 List and number of living donors to include all types: (paired exchange, regional, altruistic, adult to pediatric and pediatric to adult). Include the organ transplanted and date of donation within the past 3 years;

Lists of meeting schedules, scheduled follow-up visits, and current transplant inpatient census

7 List and number of transplant patients and living donors that are currently inpatient and the location of patient (unit and floor);
8 List and number of post-transplant patients and post-donation individuals that are scheduled for follow-up visits during the survey timeframe;
9 A schedule of any multidisciplinary team meetings that will be held during the survey;
10 A schedule of any selection committee meetings that will be held during the survey;
11 A schedule of any QAPI committee meetings that will be held during the survey;

List of organ recovery and organ offers

12 List and number of all instances where the transplant program's own recovery team recovered the donor organ for an intended recipient at their program within the last 3 years; In each instance, include the name of the transplant recipient. [If the transplant program recovers all of the deceased donor organs for a given program type, a separate list is not needed. The recipient records can be used for this sample.];
13 List and number of the organs that the transplant program received offers for within the past 3 years and declined, and the reason for the declination/UNOS decline code;

Program administration: Policies, procedures, personnel, and QAPI manuals requested for review, administrative/contracts

1 An organizational chart of the transplant program;
2 The hospital and transplant programs written agreement with their designated organ procurement organization;
3 Any contracts with external parties that the hospital or transplant program have for services relevant to transplantation including but not limited to anesthesiology, blood banking, dialysis services (inpatient or outpatient), histocompatibility (HLA) or immunology laboratory, infectious disease, internal medicine, living donor including paired exchange, regional, altruistic, adult to pediatric, or pediatric to adult donors), nursing, pathology, radiology, or surgery;

Personnel

4 List of all transplant-associated professional personnel and their titles

Table 5.3 (*Continued*)

5	The curricula, training plan, and/or training schedule for personnel (agenda, dates, evidence of attendance);
6	On-call schedule for transplant surgeons and transplant physicians for the past 30 days (includes transplant surgeon's distance and time from home to program. Does anyone have other program affiliations?)
Clinical Policies and Procedures	
7	Patient selection criteria (transplant and living donor) provide the criteria that your program uses to select patients for transplant and living donation
8	Organ recovery and organ receipt policy for ABO and other vital data verification
9	Living donor recovery for ABO and other vital data verification
10	Transplant recipient patient management for evaluation, donation, and discharge planning phases
11	Living donor patient management for evaluation, donation, and discharge planning phases
12	Waitlist management policy
13	Informed consent policy for recipients (includes associated forms)
14	Informed consent policy for living donors (includes associated forms)
15	Ongoing communication with patients and dialysis centers (informing patient and dialysis centers of patient's listing status)
Education information, policies, and procedures	
16	A copy of the written material that is distributed to potential transplant recipients and living donors to explain the selection criteria (if different from no. 7);
17	Any written educational materials used pre- and post-transplant for transplant recipients
18	Any written educational materials used pre- and post-donation for living donors
QAPI	
19	The written copy of the quality assessment and performance improvement (QAPI) program for the transplant program;
20	Any QAPI reports, records, and minutes of QAPI committee meetings, or consultation reports about the QAPI program;
21	Log of any reported adverse events for the past 12 months and corresponding documentation of the investigation and analysis of those events and any follow-up action taken.

these citations concern failures to meet volume or outcome requirements. A condition-level deficiency will put a hospital on a 90-day termination track and is not a situation that can be addressed through a "plan of correction (PoC)." A resurvey of the program will occur within 45 calendar days of the survey, provided the response on the CMS-2567 makes a credible allegation of compliance.

A standard-level deficiency is cited when the center has failed to meet one or several of the elements or standards necessary to meet a CoP. Determination of whether noncompliance is at the standard or condition level depends on the nature (how severe, how dangerous, how critical, etc.) and extent (how prevalent, how many, how pervasive, how often, etc.) of the lack of compliance. It is possible for the hospital to have several

Table 5.4 Elements to be included when submitting an acceptable plan of correction (PoC) to CMS in response to citations on the CMS-2567

- The plan for correcting each specific deficiency cited;
- Efforts to address improving the processes that led to the deficiency cited;
- The procedure for implementing the acceptable PoC for each deficiency cited;
- A completion date for correction of each deficiency cited;
- A description demonstrating how the hospital has incorporated systemic improvement actions into its quality assessment and performance improvement program in order to prevent the likelihood of the deficient practice from reoccurring;
- Procedures for monitoring and tracking to ensure that the plan of correction is in compliance with the regulatory requirements; and
- The title of the person responsible for implementing the acceptable PoC.

standard-only deficiencies yet still be found in overall compliance with the CoP as long as appropriate steps are taken to correct the deficiencies.

A PoC to address the areas cited must be submitted utilizing the CMS-2567 form within 10 calendar days of receipt of the report. CMS requires that specific elements are included in the PoC. The elements are listed in Table 5.4. Dates for the corrections to be completed for standard- or element-level deficiencies need to be no later than 45 calendar days from the date of the letter informing the center of the survey results. Dates for completion of correction for condition-level deficiencies must be within 180 calendar days. The PoC is submitted to the state's regulatory health agency.

Preparation for a survey

In order to be ready for a CMS survey, all members of the transplant team need to be educated regarding the actual requirements to comply with the regulations. Periodic reviews of the regulations should occur on a regular basis through staff meetings and other routinely occurring forums. As the time nears for a resurvey, staff should receive a "refresher course" on the survey process. It is important to encourage team members to remain calm, respectful, and "user friendly" in their interactions with surveyors. The goal should be to promote a positive, helpful environment which will enable surveyors to quickly find what they request. A cooperative and respectful attitude on the part of transplant team members ultimately enables the surveyors to perform their responsibilities in a timely manner and promotes a positive experience for all participants.

In addition to ongoing education for the team, it is helpful to have regulatory knowledge be a part of the annual competency training for new staff members. The education should include a review of how regulations may

Table 5.5 UNOS/CMS checklist

- Two ABO verifications prior to listing
- ABO verification at the time of surgery
- Compliance with removal from waitlist within 24 h of transplant or notification of death
- Compliance with notifying patients after removal from the waitlist within 10 business days for reasons other than transplant or death
- Compliance with multiple listing policy
- Compliance with data submission to UNOS of 95% forms submitted within 90 days of expected date, 100% within 6 months of expected date
- Completion of patient education checklist
- Completion of authorization to disclose protected health information
- Completion of surgical consent

play a specific part in their role within the program. For example, social workers must recognize that CMS requires patients receive a psychosocial evaluation prior to listing. Surveyors will check the date on the evaluation and the date for listing to ensure the listing occurred after the evaluation. If circumstances such as an urgent medical situation do not allow for this evaluation, a note attesting to that fact must be documented in the patient record in order to avoid a deficiency citation. If recommendations are made by social workers or by other multidisciplinary team members, surveyors will look in the medical record for evidence of follow-up actions addressing those recommendations.

Items routinely requested by the surveyor should be a placed in tabbed binders which are assembled for each transplant program. It is helpful to keep current as many documents as possible in order to produce this information in an accurate and timely manner. Individuals who would be assigned to "run the lists" for the various categories outlined need to be familiar with this task utilizing the transplant database or any other source identified for this task. Surveyors will be awaiting these lists to choose those patients whose charts they will audit, as well as which personnel they will interview. They will expect this list to be generated as quickly as possible, and significant delays in providing this information may actually result in a citation.

Another strategy to remain "survey ready" is to develop an audit tool that allows a "real-time" review of charts to determine whether documentation is evident which meets UNOS and CMS requirements. An example of an audit tool is presented in Table 5.5. Use of an audit tool helps to ensure that no chart fails to document that the patient received the appropriate education, consent, multidisciplinary care and safety processes required by regulatory agencies.

Most commonly cited deficiencies

CMS representatives state that based on 958 standard surveys, the most commonly cited deficiencies surround the requirements involved with ABO confirmations, informed consent process, evidence of multidisciplinary team involvement, patient education, and with requirements associated with QAPI activities [1].

The assessment of QAPI activities is a particular area of focus for surveyors and is discussed in more detail in Chapter 8. In a resource guide developed for transplant surveyors, there is detailed information on the various elements the surveyors will use to determine whether the transplant program meets the QAPI CoP or whether there may be standard-level deficiencies—this is found in Appendix 7.

Process for termination of Medicare certification

Any condition-level deficiency, as well as any circumstance found to create "immediate jeopardy," requires CMS to initiate termination of Medicare certification for the specific organ transplant program cited. CMS will give 210 days for a transplant program to come into compliance because of volume or outcomes contingent upon the submission of an acceptable PoC. This deadline gives a program the time necessary to affect the SRTR outcome data which is critical to the CMS approval process. If, however, the program cannot come into compliance, within the 210-day timeframe, termination will take effect. The transplant program can appeal this decision; however, termination is not delayed pending the appeal. There is also no appeal process if the application for mitigating factors has been denied. In addition to the CMS termination process, the OPTN/UNOS also has a termination process which will be discussed later in this chapter.

Mitigating factors

If a center has been given a condition-level citation, it has the option of applying for mitigating factors. What are mitigating factors? Examples of mitigating factors are highlighted in the list:

- *Extent and nature of outcome measures failure*—CMS will look at how long a program's outcomes have been below standard, the extent to which the outcomes are below standard, and whether there are unusual risk factors in the program's patient population that have contributed to below-standard outcomes.
- *Access-to-care issues*—CMS will consider if the elimination of a program will cause access to care issues for the local patient population or impact the use of organs that are procured from the local area.

- *Factors beyond the control of the hospital*—These factors would include natural disaster or changes in key physicians or surgeons.
- *Quality improvement and management interventions*—CMS will take into account if the program has performed a root-cause analysis (RCA) and embarked on performance improvement or management intervention activities. They will also consider if these activities have had a positive effect on outcomes and whether enough time has elapsed to impact the SRTR outcome data [2].

A formal written request must be submitted within 10 calendar days from the notification date on the letter accompanying the CMS-2567 form to apply for mitigating factors. Additional explanatory materials and data must be submitted within 30 calendar days from the date of the survey results letter. The application for mitigating factors usually involves trying to defend volume or outcome deficiencies. The process to apply for mitigating factors is a totally separate process from the obligation to submit a PoC within 10 days of receipt of the CMS-2567 form. An outline of the process for applying for mitigating factors is located on the CMS website at http://www.cms.gov/Medicare/Provider-Enrollment-and-Certification/CertificationandComplianc/Downloads/ConsiderationofMitigatingFactors.pdf

Systems Improvement Agreement

If CMS determines that the mitigating factors submitted are not sufficient to be approved, but has determined there is substantial commitment and evidence of actions to improve quality assessment activities, to make personnel additions or other process improvement steps, in some instances a Systems Improvement Agreement (SIA) will be offered to the hospital. The SIA is a legal contract between the Hospital and CMS that binds the hospital to engage in a rigorous series of improvement activities to address deficiencies in compliance with the CoPs. The agreement grants the hospital additional time to make substantial improvements to their transplant program and generally involves a 12-month period with a possible extension of 6 months. Failure to engage in the agreement results in loss of Medicare certification. Engagement in the contract is with the understanding that the hospital will waive any appeal rights it may have, should CMS terminate the hospital's participation of the transplant program with Medicare.

The terms of each contract may vary to some degree, but the basic elements are summarized in Table 5.6. It will likely include the engagement of a peer review team comprised of a surgeon, medical physician, transplant administrator, transplant coordinator, social worker, and quality coordinator. Individuals comprising the team need to be qualified relative to

Table 5.6 Basic elements of a Systems Improvement Agreement

- Delisting and transferring patients if necessary
- Patient notification of services during the SIA period
- Identification of peer review team
- Onsite visit of peer review team
- Root-cause analysis (RCA) plan
- Written RCA report and action plan
- On-site consultant
- Comparitive effectiveness analysis of key policies and protocols
- Staffing analysis
- Report graft failure or patient deaths
- Quarterly outcome data

experience working with the specific organ program under review. The proposed team member's credentials will be evaluated by CMS representatives and be officially approved to perform the survey.

The peer review team will visit the facility within a timeframe established in the SIA and conduct a review that entails a specific scope which is outlined in the contract. In particular, the group will examine the RCA performed by the transplant center reviewing all patient deaths or graft failures. Careful attention will be paid to confirm that the conclusions of the RCA are validated in the review of the patient records. In addition, the peer review team will conduct interviews with the transplant team members in order to determine appropriate expertise, capability, and sufficient staffing levels. Policies and protocols will be examined and the adequacy of the QAPI program will be analyzed. The QAPI program must reflect evidence of success in tracking internal information, identifying issues, analyzing outcomes, and making effective changes to improve performance in ways which will result in sustained improvements.

Following the peer review team's visit, a formal written report will be provided to the transplant center. This report remains confidential and is not provided to CMS; rather a verbal briefing will be conveyed by each member of the review team on a conference-call basis. During this call, members of the transplant program are in a "listen-only" mode and questions or comments can only be made by participants representing CMS and local state regulatory representatives. Following the call, the transplant center must develop an "action plan" to address the deficiencies and recommendations made by the peer review team. The action plan should outline the specific steps to correct each problem, primary individual accountable, expected outcome or improvement, and time line to accomplish the action. The action plan is also due for submission to CMS within a defined timeframe outlined in the SIA.

Additional requirements usually found within the SIA include an analysis of the staffing in the program relative to the need for additional personnel or training, as well as a systematic review of job descriptions and tasks assigned. A quality consultant must also be retained by the center for time periods generally ranging from 4 to 10 days onsite each month. The scope of the consultant's role is also outlined in the SIA and includes a variety of functions such as ensuring that the action plan is fully implemented with sustainable measures and that the QAPI program is robust and fully engages all of the transplant team members and representatives from hospital administration.

During the course of the SIA, monthly telephone calls are conducted with members of the transplant team, the quality consultant, and CMS representatives. Reports are given concerning progress in meeting target dates on the action plan as well as activities surrounding QAPI initiatives. Written updates and analysis on newly transplanted patients and any patient deaths or graft failures are provided in periodic reports. Near the conclusion of the SIA, the progress made to date on the action plan must be submitted and should reflect that the hospital has substantially implemented all the elements. A second visit from the peer review team may be required as part of the SIA agreement. A subset of the group may be approved to return at which time they will re-examine those areas noted to be deficient in their initial visit. They will look for evidence of improvement to program operations, personnel changes, policy revisions, QAPI activities, and at any other areas of concern they noted in their first visit. Another verbal report will be given on a conference call to CMS representatives and with transplant personnel in a 'listen-only" mode.

Based on a review of the progress made on the "action plan;" report of the second visit (if required) by the peer review team; and overall evidence of improvements that are substantial, implemented, continuing, and institutionalized, CMS will declare the program as having met approval based on mitigating factors. If CMS believes the improvements are not sustained, they can remove the approval with prior notice and an opportunity to reply.

Of note for those programs offered the SIA option is the substantial financial commitment that this process will require. For some hospitals, it may be financially prohibitive to provide the considerable funding associated with hiring the peer review team; quality consultant; and additions of surgical, medical, nursing, social work, and other healthcare personnel necessary to meet recommendations. According to data by Johns Hopkins University, the direct cost of an SIA involving liver transplant was $250,000, and with lost hospital and professional revenue, it totaled over $10 million dollars [3]. After carefully weighing all aspects involved in the SIA process, for some programs, the very difficult decision is made to close the program for a temporary period and for others the closure may be permanent.

Future trends for CMS surveys

As a result of the experiences gathered by surveyors since the publication of the CoPs in 2007, changes will be occurring in certain areas of the survey process [4]. The changes address the following areas:

- Off-site desk reviews for re-approvals of combined programs such as heart–lung and pancreas which are often low volume.
- Provision of additional outcome data to surveyors and tools to provide a better understanding of the link between data and potential quality issues.
- Maximizing opportunities to allow for direct observations of care while onsite.
- Targeted review of policies and procedures.
- A review of OPO agreements and other contracts when findings support these actions.
- The sample size for chart reviews will be scaled back relative to the number of programs to be reviewed.
- Interview questions for patients and staff will be targeted to focus on quality issues.
- Personnel record review will concentrate on areas not covered by the hospital credentialing process.
- The QAPI review with be revised and will occur earlier in the survey process, be data driven, and will guide questions and observations.

UNOS regulations

As the OPTN contractor, UNOS has established policies and bylaws which member organizations must follow in order to ensure equitable distribution of organs and to engender confidence in the national organ allocation system. Member organizations are OPOs, transplant hospitals, and histocompatibility laboratories. For this discussion, however, transplant center regulations and compliance will be the focus.

First, it is important to understand the policies and bylaws that transplant programs must adhere to. The bylaws have been established by the OPTN and cover membership and personnel requirements for the various organ transplant programs. They have recently been rewritten in a more organized and simpler fashion as mentioned in Chapter 1 and can be found on the OPTN website at http://optn.transplant.hrsa.gov/policiesAndBylaws/bylaws.asp. Samples of program applications and personnel change forms are now found on-line in the Evaluation Plan section of the UNOS website. A request for these forms for completion by the transplant program must be made to the Membership Department at UNOS, and they will send an electronic version.

The policies are also undergoing a major rewrite. These policies deal with how organs are allocated, packaged, and accepted. Also included are policies involving living donation, data submission requirements, transmissible diseases, and transplantation of non-resident aliens. The policies important to transplant programs are summarized in Table 5.7. To monitor compliance with the bylaws and policies, UNOS has set up onsite surveys as well as desk audits. The onsite audit process occurs every 3 years and desk audits are done to monitor the follow-up actions on deficiencies cited from onsite surveys or from policy violations.

The onsite surveys occur with several weeks notice. UNOS sends a list of patients for each organ group that has been either listed or transplanted to the transplant center and requests specific documentation for each patient.

Some of the data requested may be

- documentation of addition or removal from the waitlist;
- documentation of timely removal from the waitlist after transplantation or death;
- documentation of two ABO verifications prior to listing;
- documentation of patient notification within 10 days of listing or de-listing;
- documentation of the ability to double list;
- documentation of verification of donor and recipient ABO prior to implant;
- Verification of social security numbers and date of birth.

The onsite survey consists of a survey team visiting centers and reviewing a subset of patient medical records. The team verifies that the information that was sent to UNOS via the TIEDI system matches what is documented in the patient's medical record and that the OPTN policies and bylaws were followed [5]. If a policy or bylaw violation is identified, the survey team will seek explanation from the transplant center. If the explanation is inadequate, then the team will report the policy/bylaw violation to the Membership and Professional Standards Committee (MPSC) and its Policy Compliance Subcommittee (PCSC) for review and further action. If the PCSC determines that a policy or bylaw violation has occurred, it will recommend to the full MPSC the sanctions, if any, are warranted by OPTN bylaws. These sanctions include being designated a member not in good standing or the program placed on probation, or the program "voluntarily inactivating" for a period of time. The PCSC's recommendations are considered by the MPSC and may be accepted, modified, or referred back to the PCSC.

Table 5.7 Summary of UNOS policies

Transplant centers are expected to

- remove a candidate from the waiting list within 24 h of transplantation (living or deceased donor transplant) or death.

Transplant centers are expected to

- clearly define their acceptance criteria for all organs and enter this information into the UNets system.

Transplant centers are expected to

- obtain consent from candidates prior to their being listed for expanded criteria donor kidney transplantation.

Transplant centers are expected to

- list kidney transplant candidates with accurate dialysis and laboratory data;
- maintain medical record documentation of:
  - The date a candidate started chronic maintenance dialysis
  - The date a candidate's creatinine clearance or GFR was less than or equal to 20 mL/min
- maintain documentation to support all candidate data entered into UNetsm and provide such documentation upon request.

Transplant centers are expected to

- maintain documentation of a candidate's medical urgency and provide it, upon request, for review;
- reach a cooperative agreement between other local transplant centers prior to assigning medical urgency points and maintain documentation of this agreement.

Transplant centers are expected to

- obtain consent from candidates prior to their being listed for expanded criteria donor kidney transplantation.

Transplant centers are expected to

- list all candidates at the appropriate liver status or mortality risk score and to maintain medical record documentation in support of each status listing;
- provide, upon request, medical record documentation in support of listing criteria for review.

Transplant centers are expected to

- notify the host OPO when an organ recipient is suspected to have, is confirmed positive for, or has died from a potential transmissible disease or medical condition within 24 h;
- not wait for all medical documentation before informing the host OPO and/or the OPTN patient safety system

OPOs, transplant centers, and histocompatibility laboratories are expected to

- submit their respective online forms in a timely fashion according to data submission policies established within Policy 7.0 (i.e., complete 95% of forms with a quarter;
- complete 100% of forms within 6 months of their expected date). A transplant center will follow-up with transplant recipients until the recipient's death or re-transplantation.;

Transplant centers are required to

- submit follow-up information about living donors to Tiedi® at 6 months, 1 year, and 2 years following donation on the appropriate living donor follow-up (LDF) form.

Transplant centers are expected to

- ensure that each living donor is ABO typed on two separate occasions prior to the donation;

Table 5.7 (*Continued*)

- ensure that each living donor whose initial subtype test indicates the donor is non-A1 or non-A1B is ABO subtyped a second time. Blood samples for first and second test must be taken on separate occasions. Only allocate using subtype when both subtypings have the same result;
- maintain written documentation that the living donor's ABO was entered and verified by two separate individuals reviewing both of the source documents from each ABO typing.

Recovery transplant centers are expected to
- include language on living donor consent forms that indicates that vessels may be used for transplant;
- only use living donor vessels for implantation or modification of a solid organ transplant for the original recipient;
- designate a person to monitor and maintain information on all donor vessels;
- follow requirements of Policy 12 7.10.2 for any stored vessels;
- notify the OPTN of extra vessel use or disposal.

Transplant programs to report all instances of living donor deaths and failure of the living donor's native organ function within 72 h of knowledge of such event
- for kidney donors, this includes the initiation of dialysis.

Transplant programs are expected to notify UNOS when any regulatory agency takes a final adverse action against the transplant hospital
- in writing;
- within 10 business days after the OPO receives notification of the final adverse action;
- provide all documents relating to final adverse actions to UNOS.

Transplant programs are expected to address each of the following requirements in their program coverage plan:
- The program's ability to have transplant surgeons and transplant physicians available 365 days a year, 24 hours a day, 7 days a week
- That the program provides candidates with a written summary of the program coverage plan when the candidates are listed
- That the program provides candidates with a written summary of the program coverage plan when there are significant program or personnel changes
- That transplant surgeons and transplant physicians on call for the program may not simultaneously be on call for another hospital's transplant program that is more than 30 miles away
- That a transplant surgeon or transplant physician is readily available in a timely manner to
  - Facilitate organ acceptance
  - Facilitate organ procurement
  - Facilitate organ transplantation
  - Address
- That the primary transplant surgeon and primary transplant physician are not designated as the primary transplant surgeon or physician for a program at another transplant hospital unless both hospitals have additional transplant surgeons and for the programs in question

Transplant programs are expected to submit the program's written coverage plan to UNOS
- with every key personnel change, new transplant program, and new transplant hospital member application;
- upon request from UNOS staff.

(*continued*)

Table 5.7 (*Continued*)

Transplant programs are expected to
- provide candidates with a written summary of the program coverage plan when the candidates are listed;
- provide candidates with a written summary of the program coverage plan when there are significant program or personnel changes. Significant changes include
  - change in primary transplant surgeon or physician
  - becoming a single-surgeon or single-physician program
  - being able to again provide 365/24/7 coverage after previously being a single-surgeon or single-physician program
  - any other major programmatic changes that the program feels will impact or alter patients' ability to receive transplant services
  - informing patients if staffed by a single surgeon or physician

Transplant programs are expected to notify UNOS in writing when designating a new primary surgeon or primary physician, or reinstating a previously designated primary surgeon or primary physician. Written notice must:
- be sent to your regional application-related contact;
- be received by UNOS within 7 business days after the program is informed of the change.

Source: Data from the UNOS Evaluation Plan September 1, 2012.

The clinical performance of a transplant center is also monitored by the OPTN. When SRTR data reveal that a center is performing with less than expected outcomes of either patient or graft survival, the center is referred to the members of the Performance Analysis and Improvement Subcommittee (PAIS) of the MPSC.

As mentioned earlier, UNOS employs the peer review process and, as such, guarantees the confidentiality of its member organizations. The identity of the member in question is blinded to the committees unless, of course, the MPSC's review requires a subsequent formal disciplinary proceeding. The recommendations of the MPSC ultimately will be voted on by the UNOS Board of Directors.

UNOS also conducts two other types of peer visits apart from the survey process:
- Investigative peer visits which are used to identify the problem or issue at an organization, including potential patient safety issues.
- Advisory peer visits that provide feedback to the member on committee reviews and provide a way for the committee to monitor the member's improvement efforts. Typically, advisory peer visits are conducted for transplant programs with lower than expected outcomes.

UNOS is currently working with CMS to identify requirements that overlap and to come to some agreement on how the agencies can work together in order to facilitate regulatory oversight of transplant centers. Some progress is being made in regard to sharing survey information in order to reduce redundancy, and talks are underway to develop one survey process. This will greatly reduce the compliance burden of transplant programs in the future.

Joint Commission

TJC accredits and certifies healthcare programs in the United States in order to assure the public that the organization meets certain quality and performance standards. They have traditionally surveyed hospital in-patient units and other areas within the hospital; however, TJC has recently begun surveying ambulatory settings, which includes transplant clinics. The major areas that TJC reviews and questions to ask are as follows:

- Emergency management—Is there a disaster plan in place? Are there fire extinguishers and have they been inspected within the prescribed period of time? Are there clearly labeled emergency exits?
- Infection control—Are there hand santizers outside of key areas and clinic rooms? Are there gloves, masks, and gowns available if needed?
- Medication management—Are crash carts inspected regularly? Are medications being stored in a refrigerator and if so, is the temperature continuously monitored? Are medications all within shelf-life?
- Provision of care—Are medical supplies available in all clinic rooms and are they within shelf-life? Is there a process for patients to sign in for their appointment that ensures confidentiality? Is there a process for patients to know what they need to do to follow-up after the clinic visit, i.e., return appointment or further testing?
- Record of care—Are verbal orders documented properly? Are physician orders signed, timed, and dated? Is there a plan of care in the medical record? Are medical records stored in a secured area with controlled access? Are medical records in use kept in areas to ensure confidentiality?
- Right of the individual—Are patient consents signed and dated in the medical record?

The site survey for the transplant clinic occurs during the site survey for the hospital and may take 3 to 4 hours for the surveyor to complete their inspection. The administrator and a clinic nurse/coordinator should be available for the surveyor to show them the clinic and areas of interest, to answer questions, and to go through the patient records. The surveyor will select several patient charts and will want to examine them for the items mentioned above. Any identified deficiencies will not be mentioned until the exit conference at the completion of the entire hospital inspection.

The Joint Commission certification process for destination ventricular assist device (VAD) programs

The oversight of a ventricular assist device (VAD) program is often included as a part of the responsibilities for the transplant administrator associated with a heart transplant program. VAD services are now routinely offered in conjunction with heart transplant programs as a "bridge therapy" to sustain patients during the wait time for a donor organ. In some instances when patients are not suitable for transplant, they are evaluated for a VAD as a permanent or destination type of therapy. In 2007, Medicare established TJC as the deeming authority to establish guidelines and standards of care for patients having a VAD implanted as a permanent form of therapy. Following the publication of the guidelines, centers were required to meet the certification requirements by March of 2009 or lose reimbursement for patients with Medicare funding. The process was part of TJC disease-specific care (DSC) standards certification, and VAD programs were further delineated as falling under the category of advanced disease-specific certification. Information regarding the DSC standards and the process for obtaining certification for advanced disease-specific programs can be found at http://www.jointcommission.org/certification/diseasespecific_care.aspx. Examples of other programs in this category include lung volume reduction surgery (LVRS), stroke centers, chronic kidney disease, and heart failure. In order for hospitals to receive the advanced disease-specific VAD for destination therapy certification, they must meet the requirements outlined in the DSC certification manual. In addition, they must also:

1 be providing VAD destination therapy to an adult population;
2 have facilities with the infrastructure to support VAD placements as evidenced by adequate staffing and facilities to perform and recover patients after cardiac surgery;
3 be an active continuous member of a national, audited registry for mechanically assisted circulatory support devices that requires submission of health data on VAD destination therapy patients from the date of implantation throughout the remainder of their lives;
4 include a board-certified cardiac surgeon who meets the following volume requirements:
   a Placed 10 VADs in the last 36 months with current activity in the last 12 months. If a surgeon on the team has not placed 10 VADs during the required time period, the volume requirements can be met by including artificial heart placements for no more than 50% of the total volume.
   b The volume requirement is effective at the time the application is submitted to TJC. It is considered over a rolling time period effective at the time of application or renewal.

The evaluation of the program will be made using the standards in the DSC certification manual. The program must demonstrate conformity with clinical practice guidelines or evidence-based practice that includes the VAD-specific requirements that are integrated with the disease-specific care requirements. All certified VAD programs will be required to comply with the Phase I requirements for performance measurement until standardized performance measures have been identified. As part of Phase I requirements for performance measurement, programs are required to collect and analyze data on at least four performance measures related to or identified in clinical practice guidelines for each program or service. Measures selected by the program or service should be evidence based, relevant, valid, and reliable. TJC will not be prescriptive during Stage I regarding which specific measures are to be implemented; the emphasis will be on the use of performance measures for improving care. The standards require the DSC program or service to demonstrate that it

- routinely applies the cycle for performance improvements to identify and address improvement opportunities;
- implements a plan for improvement and graphically depicts measurement results over time to demonstrate improvement in the measured areas;
- reviews the effectiveness of the interventions implemented in response to improvement opportunities identified by the measurement activity.

Programs apply through an electronic process to TJC to receive consideration for certification of their VAD destination program. The application is a two-part electronic document and requires organizational demographic information and preferred month of onsite review. References used for establishing the clinical practice guidelines are requested and the specifics including rationale, for the four performance measures utilized by the program. The information provided is analyzed in advance of the onsite visit and provides surveyors with the organization's current strengths and growth opportunities. Upon acceptance of the application, TJC will provide the center with dates for a 1.5-day onsite survey.

Preparation for a successful survey requires an intensive systematic approach and the involvement of all members of the VAD program team [6]. At the start of the survey, an overview PowerPoint presentation can be provided which highlights the program's history, staff, and the four performance measures the program has identified to analyze for improvement. Typical survey activities include interviewing the medical and nursing staff for the VAD program; nurse managers for the operating room, ICU, and step-down unit; patients that may be in the hospital or returning for a clinic visit; and nursing staff that are assigned to their care. A visit to clinical areas involved with the care of VAD patients is conducted. A substantial part of the survey entails performing tracers on charts for inpatients and those discharged following VAD implantation. A tracer may reveal a patient having services in areas of the hospital that may also be visited by the surveyor. Questions may be asked of staff in these areas regarding how they would care for a VAD patient in their department. Common areas of documentation that are reviewed as part of the tracer include

- consents;
- selection committee notes;
- social work notes;
  - operative notes;
  - inpatient order sets and readmission order sets;
  - evidence that antibiotics were administered per protocol in the OR;
  - nursing notes and evidence of patient teaching regarding dressing changes, discharge preparation, and evidence of patient having met transfer criteria from ICU to floor and discharge criteria;
  - home environment safety check completed.

In addition to performing tracers, the surveyor will conduct a personnel record review for surgeons, medical directors, VAD-trained nurses, and clinical engineers. The records must reflect appropriate credentialing and evidence of training for care of VAD patients and documentation of ongoing education and competency. At the conclusion of the survey, the team will hear the surveyor's impressions and the decision with regard to receiving TJC certification. The certification is valid for 2 years with ongoing submission of performance measures and an off-site intracycle review in 1 year. Subsequent surveys are likely more rigorous than the initial one, and VAD programs must devote the appropriate staff to maintain the data registry, quality assessment, and performance improvement activities and ensure patient safety in the outpatient setting.

References

1 Tritz K. 2012. CMS, Part 2 – The Survey Process, Policies and Future Activities. April, 2012. Presentation at UNOS Transplant Management Forum.

2 CMS. Process For Requesting Consideration of Mitigating Factors in CMS' Determination of Medicare Approval of Organ Transplant Centers. http://www.cms.gov/Medicare/Provider-Enrollment-and-Certification/CertificationandComplianc/Downloads/ConsiderationofMitigatingFactors.pdf. Accessed October 4, 2013.

3 Sullivan B. Beyond CMS Certification: Mitigating Factors Application and Systems Improvement Applications. April, 2012. Presentation at UNOS Transplant Management Forum.

4 Pizzolato K. Future CMS Surveys – What to Expect. April 2013. Presentation at UNOS Transplant Management Forum.
5 UNOS. Staying Between the Lines. 2010. UNOS Update. July/August: p. 23.
6 Lockard K, Weimer A, O'Shea G, et al. The Joint Commission's disease – specific care certification for destination therapy ventricular assist devices. *Prog Transplant.* 2010;20(2):155–162.

CHAPTER 6
Transplant Finance

Lisa Norris
Transplant Leadership Institute LLC, San Antonio, TX, USA

Hospitals are anticipating dramatic shifts in reimbursement as the national healthcare legislation becomes actualized. Accountable care organizations (ACOs) are being created, and hospitals have been acquiring physician practices in order to broaden their referral bases. It is now more important than ever for the transplant enterprise to demonstrate that it is cost-effective and profitable. No longer can a program assume that it contributes a positive margin to the hospital—it must be proven in this era of extreme fiscal belt-tightening. This chapter gives a brief history to the way programs are reimbursed and examines the financial aspects that are unique to transplant programs, with special emphasis on financial monitoring methods, cost reporting, and financial performance.

Revenue sources

There are several revenue sources for a transplant program, the most notable being Medicare, Medicaid, and private insurers.

Medicare

Medicare is a federally funded program that came into existence in 1965 and provides health insurance to those aged 65 and older. In 1972, Medicare was expanded to include the disabled and those with end-stage renal disease. Medicare has several parts:

- Part A—Covers in-patient services, outpatient diagnostic services, and extended care after hospitalization
- Part B—Covers physician services and outpatient services
- Part C—This is the Medicare plus choice program or Medicare advantage plans
- Part D—covers prescription drugs for Medicare recipients

Medicare was amended in 1983 to include the prospective payment system for reimbursement and established the diagnosis-related groups

Transplant Administration, First Edition. Edited by Lisa Norris.

Companion website: www.wiley.com/go/norris/transplantadmin

Table 6.1 Transplant crosswalk from DRG to MS DRG

Type of transplant	DRG	MS-DRG
Heart transplant or implant of heart assist system w MCC	103	001
Heart transplant or implant of heart assist system w/o MCC	103	002
Liver transplant w MCC or intestinal transplant	480	005
Liver transplant w/o MCC	480	006
Lung transplant	495	007
Simultaneous pancreas/kidney transplant	512	008
Pancreas transplant	513	010
Kidney transplant	302	652

MCC, major complications and comorbidities.

(DRGs) [1]. In 2008, there was further refinement in the DRGs to include medical severity which are termed MS-DRGs. The DRGs and MS-DRGs for transplant patients are summarized in Table 6.1. Payments to hospitals for each DRG include a hospital-specific DRG base rate multiplied by a DRG assigned weight. The DRG base rate is adjusted for different wage levels and includes an amount for capital costs and, for qualifying hospitals, an additional amount may be given for serving a disproportionate share of low-income persons, for costs associated with medical education programs, or for the hospital being located in a rural area.

Up until 1992, Medicare reimbursed physicians on a reasonable and customary basis; however, it then implemented the resource-based relative value system (RBRVS) which reimbursed physicians on a flat fee per visit [2]. Medicare has also been amended to reimburse outpatient services based on Ambulatory Payment Classification system or APC. There are several items that are important to know about Medicare, as far as transplant is concerned. Medicare provides:

- coverage for patients who are aged 65, disabled (24 or more months), or have end-stage renal disease;
- coverage the month the patient receives a kidney transplant if the patient does not already have Medicare;
- coverage only to those transplanted in a Medicare-approved facility;
- immunosuppressive drug coverage for 3 years post-transplant only if the patient is transplanted in a Medicare-approved facility;
- drug coverage under Part D; however, there is no coverage when costs fall between $2970 and $4700 (donut hole). Additional help is available for those with low incomes;
- coverage for simultaneous kidney/pancreas and pancreas after kidney transplant;
- coverage for living donors;
- additional reimbursement via the Medicare cost report, which is discussed later in this chapter.

Medicaid

Medicaid was established in 1965 to provide health insurance coverage for those who are medically indigent or unable to pay for medical services. It is a dually funded program between the states and the federal government and administered by each individual state. Eligibility for Medicaid varies from state to state; however, there are basically two categories of "need" that states recognize. First, there is the categorically needy classification which the states are required to cover in order to receive federal funding. Included are low-income families with children, children, pregnant women, seniors, and individuals with disabilities. The second group is the medically needy, which refers to those who are Medicaid eligible because they have sizable medical costs and their income is too high to qualify in categorically needy category. This classification is not offered in every state, but it allows individuals to "spend down" their income with their medical expenses. The purpose is to bring the income down to the federal poverty level (FPL) in order to qualify for Medicaid. Effective January 2014, individuals under 65 years of age with income below 133% of the FPL will be eligible for Medicaid. This will allow low-income adults without children to be covered through Medicaid in every state without need for a waiver, and parents of children will be eligible at a uniform income level across all states.

As far as transplantation benefits, it is up to each state to determine whether Medicaid will pay for organ transplant. Usually, it involves a lengthy approval process and even if a particular organ transplant is covered, there may be qualifying conditions and criteria that apply. For example, some states will not cover living donor liver transplants or heart transplants for patients who are over the age of 65. Most states will also not cover a transplant that takes place in a different state.

Private insurers

In the 1930s and 1940s, there was a push to create compulsory health insurance under the Roosevelt and Truman administrations. However, this legislation was defeated, which allowed the growth of voluntary and private health insurance industry in the United States [3]. The first commercial insurance plan was Blue Cross, and subsequently employers began to offer health insurance as a benefit to attract workers. In the 1990s, healthcare costs rose astronomically which prompted the formation of health maintenance organizations (HMOs). The purpose of these organizations was to moderate the rapid escalation of healthcare costs. Although there was much resistance of hospitals and physicians to working with HMOs, they eventually gained wide acceptance. There are several items that are important to know about these organizations:

- Managed care organizations (MCOs) use utilization review to control costs. This review is usually performed by trained nurses who may deny

claims of services which they think are unnecessary. Utilization review can take place before care delivery, during the in-patient stay, or after the care has been delivered.
- Primary care physicians typically are used as gatekeepers to control referrals to specialists; however, this is changing within the industry.
- Enrollees are encouraged to seek treatment from only those physicians who are within their network. Currently, most allow the option of seeking care out-of-network, but patients will pay higher out-of-pocket costs.
- Case managers are employed to coordinate care of complex patients or those with chronic conditions.
- They attempt to share financial risk with hospitals or providers.

Transplant programs receive reimbursement from HMOs or MCOs through contracts that are separate from the hospital's contracts for general services—i.e., "carved out." How transplant programs specifically relate to MCOs is discussed in Chapter 7.

Organ acquisition

One of the significant business advantages distinct to transplant programs is the ability to pass pretransplant costs to the Medicare cost report. The Medicare cost report is a year-end report that determines the federal government's payment for services for Medicare beneficiaries and on average provides $4.7 million dollars of revenue to each transplant program [4]. Transplant costs that are allowable for inclusion on the cost report are organ donor and recipient costs before hospital admission for the transplant or pretransplant costs and hospital in-patient costs associated with the donor. These costs and the Medicare cost reporting rules are very difficult to comprehend for most hospital administrators, transplant administrators and physicians. Typically, a hospital reimbursement specialist assists in the process, and an outside agency (Ernest and Young, Deloitte, and others) as well as a fiscal intermediary (FI) will audit their submissions. A FI is a private company who is contracted with CMS to review hospital cost reports and determine the allowability of costs claimed. It is interesting to note that despite the external and internal review of the transplant cost report, the Office of Inspector General (OIG) in an audit of 13 transplant centers found that Medicare overpaid transplant centers in the majority of cases. The most common reasons why costs were deemed unallowable were:
- costs were not properly documented;
- costs exceeded physician salary limits;
- costs were inappropriately allocated to organ acquisition cost [5].

Violation of the False Claims Act may also apply in these OIG cases. The act states that those who knowingly submit, or cause another person or entity to submit, false claims for payment of government funds are liable for three times the government's damages plus civil penalties of $5500 to $11,000 per false claim. Under the qui tam provisions, a whistleblower may receive 15–25% of the settlement [6]. It is also recommended that any external experts who are examining Medicare cost report data be hired by the hospital's legal team and as such be under the auspices of attorney–client privilege. This protects documents from discovery and the hospital from potential governmental action. Although it is rare that an auditor would violate professional ethics, it has indeed occurred. The following case study describes a transplant qui tam case involving the cost report which further illustrates the necessity of being vigilant about transplant cost reporting.

Case study: The transplant cost report and the False Claims Act

In 2003, Sharp Memorial Hospital in San Diego, California, agreed to pay over $6.2 million to settle a suit over Medicare Cost Report overpayments. The suit began as a whistleblower suit filed under the *qui tam* provisions of the False Claims Act by a transplant coordinator. The transplant coordinator was given information about the cost report submissions and was concerned about items included in the transplant cost report as she was knowledgeable about what was allowable. She went to the hospital administration to voice her concerns, but was rebuffed. She then filed a suit under the False Claims Act *Qui Tam* provision and alleged that the hospital included items that were not reimbursable, such as staff salaries, medical director fees, laboratory costs, and square footage. Although the hospital denied any wrongdoing, a settlement was reached and the coordinator and her attorneys received $1.2 million as a share of the recovery under the settlement. Encouraging a culture of compliance and taking employee's concerns seriously is the lesson learned in this case.

Source: www.justice.gov/opa/pr/2003/March/03_civ_139.htm

Organ acquisition costs are paid by Medicare to certified organ transplant centers on a reasonable cost basis. These are separate from the DRG payment to the hospital for the in-patient stay and the physician fees associated with the transplant. It is important to establish organ acquisition cost centers in the transplant program so that costs can be accumulated by organ and then by pretransplant or post-transplant. In addition, having a transplant administration cost center is also beneficial, and it can be allocated based on the volume of organs of each type of organ transplanted. The cost report preparation will be less complicated by having these cost centers in place. So what is included in organ acquisition costs?

Organ acquisition is comprised of both direct and indirect costs. The direct costs are those directly related to organ acquisition. There are also indirect costs which are costs associated with overhead, such as

Table 6.2 Direct organ acquisition costs

Cost of deceased and live donor organs
Tissue typing
Donor and recipient evaluation
UNOS registry fees
Operating room and other in-patient services for the donor
Transportation and perfusion/preservation costs
Surgeon fees for procurement of cadaveric organs
Procurement services by residents not in a teaching hospital
Post-op services to living donors for any complications
Salaries of staff relating to pretransplant activities

housekeeping, administration, among others. A list of direct organ acquisition costs is summarized in Table 6.2. Some of the costs that are not allowable are disease management, travel or lodging, and research protocols. It is very important that all pretransplant costs are accumulated into the organ acquisition cost center—both private and public payors. Medicare will then pay their share of the cost based on the volume of Medicare transplants for that year. In other words, if Medicare transplants account for 50% of your total transplant volume (this includes those where Medicare is primary and secondary payor), then Medicare will pay 50% of your allowable organ acquisition cost less any revenue realized from cadaveric donors procured in-house (Figure 6.1). In addition, it must be stressed that for all pretransplant evaluation services that are purchased (such as laboratory, tissue typing, physician evaluation fees), the hospital is the payor and should have a contract for these services in place. A transplant program should pay the Medicare allowable for these purchased services—a survey of 43 transplant centers found that only 65% use Medicare rates for reimbursement [7].

The cost report

The Medicare cost report is comprised of multiple worksheets; however, those that are of particular relevance to transplant are Worksheets A, B-1, and D-4. Worksheet A of the cost report is entitled "Reclassification and Adjustment of Trial Balance of Expenses" and is used to group total provider expenses minus nonallowable expenses to arrive at net allowable expenses for allocation. The direct costs of organ acquisition should be placed on Worksheet A of the cost report. The part of Worksheet A which pertains to organ acquisition is shown in Figure 6.2.

(Organ acquisition costs × medicare ratio) – revenue for cadaveric organs

Figure 6.1 Medicare apportionment calculation.

4090 (Cont.) FORM CMS-2552-10 08-11

RECLASSIFICATION AND ADJUSTMENT OF TRIAL BALANCE OF EXPENSES					PROVIDER *CCN:*		PERIOD: FROM ________ TO ________		WORKSHEET A	
		COST CENTER DESCRIPTIONS (omit cents)	SALARIES	OTHER	TOTAL (col.1 + col. 2)	RECLASSIFI-CATIONS	RECLASSIFIED TRIAL BALANCE (col. 3 ± col. 4)	ADJUSTMENTS	NET EXPENSES FOR ALLOCATION (col. 5 ± col. 6)	
			1	2	3	4	5	6	7	
		OTHER REIMBURSABLE COST CENTERS								
94	09400	Home Program Dialysis								94
95	09500	Ambulance Services								95
96	09600	Durable Medical Equipment-rented								96
97	09700	Durable Medical Equipment-sold								97
98		Other Reimbursable (specify)								98
99		Outpatient Rehabilitation Provider (specify)								99
100	10000	Intern-Resident Service (not appvd. tchng. prgm.)								100
101	10100	Home Health Agency								101
		SPECIAL PURPOSE COST CENTERS								
105	10500	Kidney Acquisition								105
106	10600	Heart Acquisition								106
107	10700	Liver Acquisition								107
108	10800	Lung Acquisition								108
109	10900	Pancreas Acquisition								109
110	11000	Intestinal Acquisition								110
111	11100	Islet Acquisition								111
112		Other Organ Acquisition (specify)								112
113	11300	Interest Expense							- 0 -	113
114	11400	Utilization Review-snf							- 0 -	114
115	11500	Ambulatory Surgical Center (Distinct part)								115
116	11600	Hospice								116
117		Other Special Purpose (specify)								117
118		Subtotals (sum of lines 1-117)								118
		NONREIMBURSABLE COST CENTERS								
190	19000	Gift, Flower, Coffee Shop & Canteen								190
191	19100	Research								191
192	19200	Physicians' Private Offices								192
193	19300	Nonpaid Workers								193
194		Other Nonreimbursable (specify)								194
200		TOTAL (sum of lines 118-199)				- 0 -				200

Figure 6.2 Sample of Medicare cost report Worksheet A.
Source: http://www.costreportdata.com.

Table 6.3 Time study log

		STAFF WEEKLY TIME REPORT						
EMPLOYEE'S NAME: ____________								
ACQUISITION COST CENTER: __________								
WEEK OF:								
EMPLOYEE'S SIGNATURE: __________								
DATE								
	SUN	MON	TUES	WED	THUR	FRI	SAT	TOTAL
*TIME IN								
*TIME OUT								
HOURS WORKED								
ON-CALL TIME								
						TOTAL HOURS		0
		PRETRANSPLANT TIME STUDY						
	SUN	MON	TUES	WED	THUR	FRI	SAT	TOTAL
ORGAN ALLOCATION								
RECIPIENT/DONOR DATA								
COLLECTION								
MEDICAL MGMT/REVIEW								
TEACHING/COUNSELING								
DIALYSIS OUTREACH								
FINANCIAL								
ADMINISTRATIVE/CLERICAL								
BUSINESS DEVELOPMENT								
REGULATORY COMPLIANCE								
LIVING DONOR EVALUATION								
UNOS NETWORK DATA								
MEETINGS								
				TOTAL PRETRANSPLANT HOURS				0
		POST-TRANSPLANT TIME STUDY						
	SUN	MON	TUES	WED	THUR	FRI	SAT	TOTAL
TEACHING/COUNSELING								
ADMINISTRATIVE/CLERICAL								
OUTPATIENT MANAGEMENT								
IN-PATIENT ROUNDS								
OTHER								
				TOTAL POST-TRANSPLANT HOURS				0

First, only a portion of staff salaries that relate to organ acquisition activities (pretransplant) are cost reimbursed. In order to comply with Medicare regulations, transplant programs must have documentation in order to account for the time spent by staff and physicians on organ acquisition activity. Examples of these activities include nonbillable patient management, organ procurement organization (OPO) meetings, patient selection meetings, dialysis outreach, education of donors and recipients, data submission, and education. For physicians, only the time spent on pretransplant administrative tasks relating to their role as medical or surgical director would qualify to be included on the cost report. Clinical time spent with pretransplant patients is not included since physicians already bill for that time. These time studies should be filled out by staff 1 week each month. Each week chosen should rotate in order to obtain an average of the overall pretransplant time. Physicians must account for all of their administrative time. Tables 6.3 and 6.4 illustrate templates used for staff and physicians. For auditing purposes, it is also helpful if job descriptions can specify pre- or post-transplant to give further support for the allocation of coordinator time. The studies should be reviewed by the transplant administrator or transplant business manager and then filed in the event of audit.

Medicare places limits on the compensation that be written off to the cost report for medical directors based on reasonable compensation equivalents (RCEs) [8]. The method for determining RCE limits is based on physician specialty and the type of location which can be seen in Table 6.5 [9]. Most transplant programs pay for medical directorships to compensate physicians and surgeons for their administrative duties (Table 6.6). Most salaries are based on an estimation of time spent and the market rate of physician time. Most hospitals pay their physicians and

Table 6.4 Physician time study template

Monthly Physician Time Study Form
Physician Name________________
Month and Year________________

Number of Hours	Week 1	Week 2	Week 3	Week 4
QAPI				
Records review				
Community outreach/education				
Team meetings				
Living donor counseling				
Referring MD outreach				
Pretransplant on-call				
Other administrative work				
Total hours				

Monthly total hours________
I hereby certify that the services provided are accurate and true.
Physician signature________________ _______ Date_________

Table 6.5 Estimates of FTE annual average net compensation levels for cost reporting periods beginning on or after January 1, 2004*

Specialty	Nonmetropolitan	Metropolitan <1 million	Metropolitan >1 million
Total	159,800	171,400	177,200
General/Family Practice	142,500	136,700	138,700
Internal Medicine	150,200	154,100	165,600
Surgery	182,900	204,100	208,000
Pediatrics	130,900	152,100	140,600
OB/GYN	200,300	194,500	196,400
Radiology	217,600	231,100	225,300
Psychiatry	138,700	142,500	154,100
Anesthesiology	167,500	200,300	200,300
Pathology	208,000	219,500	215,700

Source: Centers for Medicare and Medicaid Services, Aug. 1, 2003 Federal Register, vol. 68, No. 148.
*All figures are rounded to the nearest $100.

surgeons at a rate equal to their current pay. However, the cost report reimbursement for these directorships is very different. For example, if a surgeon is compensated for 1000 hours per year at an hourly rate of $200 per hour or $200,000, the amount that can be reimbursed under the cost report is as follows:

RCE limit rate ($177,200/2080 hours per year) is $85.19 per hour
1000 hours × $85.19 is $85,190

So, only $85,190 should be placed on the cost report for reimbursement.

Another direct expense that merits further examination is organ procurement fees. Procurement fees may also be called standard acquisition

Table 6.6 Physician directorship duties

Attend leadership meetings with regularity
Monitor overall quality and appropriateness of care
Progress toward process improvement activities
Provide guidance and leadership for performance guidelines
Participate in strategic planning
Participate in policy formation including written documentation and procedures
Oversee clinical peer review
Oversee the plan of care
Manage internal and external relationships
Be a representative of the program or organization
Handle clinical patient complaints
Address emergency issues
Handle physician behavior and related issues

Source: http://www.mgma.com/blog/medical-director-job-description/.

Table 6.7 Surgeon procurement fees

Organ	Mean fee	Median fee
Kidney	1640	1250
Liver	4177	4000
Heart	3022	2800
Pancreas	2776	2600
Single lung	3010	3000
Double lung	2725	2875
Intestine	2615	2500

Source: 2012 American Organ Procurement Organization Annual Report.

charges (SAC fees) and are set by the organ procurement organization based on the average cost associated with of a deceased donor organ. Medicare reimburses OPOs for the cost of kidney procurement (currently set at $1250), but not for the cost related to the other organs. The OPO incorporates into the SAC fee the direct cost of procurement, salaries and benefits of staff, and administrative cost. When an organ is imported, the transplant program pays the organ acquisition fee of the nonlocal OPO in addition to the procuring physician fees and transportation. Imported organs, therefore, are at a much higher cost than locally procured organs. The mean and median of surgeon procurement fees are summarized Table 6.7 and the 2013 OPO kidney SAC fees are summarized in Appendix 8. Please note that surgeon fees for organs that are discarded are much lower than those found in Table 6.7 (typically approximately $1000 per organ). Many administrators and physicians have expressed that containing the ever-rising OPO SAC fees is frustrating. It presents a real challenge for a transplant program that operates in a competitive managed care environment since payors rarely favor an increase in rates except for a small concession for inflation. The best way to tackle escalating SAC fees is to have influence with the OPO board of directors.

Although most OPO's do not have a procurement fee for living donor organs, there is much confusion surrounding how to account for these expenses on the cost report. This is particularly true for centers participating in paired kidney exchange programs or for centers that have pediatric programs where the recipient is at one facility and the adult donor excision takes place at another facility. Medicare mandates that all donor expenses must be charged to the transplant center where the recipient receives the organ. The donor center should not account for any expenses of the donation on their cost report and should bill the recipient center for all costs associated with the donation.

Many centers have created a SAC for both deceased and living organs, which is billed to the recipient. It is interesting to note that in 2009, 20% of transplant programs reported no salaries on Worksheet A and 8% reported no direct organ acquisition expenses [10]. Obviously, this is money left on the table, and it behooves each transplant leader to meet with their reimbursement counterpart to review the cost report prior to filing.

Worksheet B series of the Medicare cost report allows for the allocation of overhead or indirect costs to patient care cost centers. These indirect costs are associated with the general of running the hospital (such as housekeeping, dietary, cafeteria, and medical records) and are allocated from the general service cost centers to the organ acquisition cost center as shown in Figure 6.3. The use of space for transplant services bears special mention. Space costs are typically allocated based on square footage, and pretransplant must be distinguished from post-transplant. This can be accomplished several ways, by using either the percentage of pretransplant patients to total patients or the pretransplant staff salaries to total salaries and applying that same percentage to the total space occupied by the transplant program including clinic. Space costs also need to be allocated among organs based on the ratio of number of transplants for particular organ to total transplants.

Worksheet D-4 (formerly D-6) provides for the computation and accumulation of organ acquisition costs and charges for Medicare-certified transplant programs. Only Medicare-certified transplant centers will be reimbursed by Medicare for organ acquisition cost. Worksheet D-4 consists of the following four parts:

- Part I—Computation of organ acquisition cost (in-patient routine and ancillary services)
- Part II—Computation of organ acquisition cost (other than that in Part I)
- Part III—Summary of costs and charges
- Part IV—Statistics [11]

Several points should be kept in mind regarding Worksheet D-4:

- Allowable charges for all pretransplant patients regardless of payor should be accumulated on Part I of the Worksheet (Figure 6.4) including all charges for living donors (pretransplant, in-patient, and post-transplant).
- Exact counts of the organs excised, organs purchased from the OPO, organs sold to the OPO, unusable organs excised, Medicare primary organs transplanted, Medicare secondary organs transplanted, and other payor transplants should be placed on Worksheet D-4 Part IV. It is important to keep accurate counts and documentation for each of these.

The expectation for the transplant administrator is not to be an expert in cost reporting, but to be familiar with the cost report and to assist the finance department in cost report preparation by ensuring that organ

08-11 FORM CMS-2552-10 4090 (Cont.)

COST ALLOCATION - STATISTICAL BASIS								PROVIDER CCN:		PERIOD: FROM ____ TO ____		WORKSHEET B-1	

	COST CENTER DESCRIPTIONS	OTHER GENERAL SERVICE (SPECIFY)	NON-PHYSICIAN ANES-THETISTS (ASGND TIME)	NURSING SCHOOL (ASSIGNED TIME)	INTERNS & RESIDENTS SALARY AND FRINGES (ASSIGNED TIME)	INTERNS & RESIDENTS PROGRAM COSTS (ASSIGNED TIME)	PARA-MEDICAL EDUCATION (ASSIGNED TIME)	SUBTOTAL	INTERN & RESIDENT COST & POST STEPDOWN ADJUSTMENTS	TOTAL	
		18	19	20	21	22	23	24	25	26	
	OTHER REIMBURSABLE COST CENTERS										
94	Home Program Dialysis										94
95	Ambulance Services										95
96	Durable Medical Equipment-Rented										96
97	Durable Medical Equipment-Sold										97
98	Other Reimbursable (specify)										98
99	Outpatient Rehabilitation Provider (specify)										99
100	Intern-Resident Service (not appvd. tchng. prgm.)										100
101	Home Health Agency										101
	SPECIAL PURPOSE COST CENTERS										
105	Kidney Acquisition										105
106	Heart Acquisition										106
107	Liver Acquisition										107
108	Lung Acquisition										108
109	Pancreas Acquisition										109
110	Intestinal Acquisition										110
111	Islet Acquisition										111
112	Other Organ Acquisition (specify)										112
115	Ambulatory Surgical Center (Distinct Part)										115
116	Hospice										116
117	Other Special Purpose (specify)										117
118	SUBTOTALS (sum of lines 1-117)										118
	NONREIMBURSABLE COST CENTERS										
190	Gift, Flower, Coffee Shop, & Canteen										190
191	Research										191
192	Physicians' Private Offices										192
193	Nonpaid Workers										193
194	Other Nonreimbursable (specify)										194
200	Cross foot adjustments										200
201	Negative cost centers										201
202	Cost to be allocated (per Worksheet B, Part I)										202
203	Unit cost multiplier (Worksheet B, Part I)										203
204	Cost to be allocated (per Worksheet B, Part II)										204
205	Unit cost multiplier (Worksheet B, Part II)										205

Figure 6.3 Example of Medicare cost report Worksheet B-1.
Source: http://www.costreportdata.com.

08-11 FORM CMS-2552-10 4090 (Cont.)

COMPUTATION OF ORGAN ACQUISITION COSTS AND CHARGES FOR HOSPITALS WHICH ARE CERTIFIED TRANSPLANT CENTERS	PROVIDER CCN: ____ OPO CCN: ____	PERIOD: FROM ____ TO ____	WORKSHEET D-4, PART I

Check applicable box:	[ ] HEART	[ ] LIVER	[ ] PANCREAS	[ ] ISLET
	[ ] KIDNEY	[ ] LUNG	[ ] INTESTINE	[ ] OTHER (specify)

PART I - COMPUTATION OF ORGAN ACQUISITION COSTS (INPATIENT ROUTINE AND ANCILLARY SERVICES)

	Computation of Inpatient Routine Service Costs Applicable to Organ Acquisition	Inpatient Routine Organ Charges		Per Diem Costs (from Wkst. D-1, Part II)	Organ Acquisition Days	Cost (col. 2 x col. 3)	
		1	D	2	3	4	
1	Adults and Pediatrics		38				1
2	Intensive Care		43				2
3	Coronary Care		44				3
4	Burn Intensive Care Unit		45				4
5	Surgical Intensive Care Unit		46				5
6	Other Special Care (specify)		47				6
7	TOTAL (sum of lines 1-6)						7

	Computation of Ancillary Service Costs Applicable to Organ Acquisition		Ratio of Cost to Charges (from Wkst. C)	Organ Acquisition Ancillary Charges	Organ Acquisition Ancillary Costs	
		C	1	2	3	
8	Operating Room	50				8
9	Recovery Room	51				9
10	Labor Room & Delivery Room	52				10
11	Anesthesiology	53				11
12	Radiology-Diagnostic	54				12
13	Radiology-Therapeutic	55				13
14	Radioisotope	56				14
15	Computed Tomography (CT) Scan	57				15
16	Magnetic Resonance Imaging (MRI)	58				16
17	Cardiac Catheterization	59				17
18	Laboratory	60				18
19	PBP Clinical Laboratory Services-Program Only	61				19
20	Whole Blood & Packed Red Blood Cells	62				20
21	Blood Storage, Processing, & Transfusing	63				21
22	IV Therapy	64				22
23	Respiratory Therapy	65				23
24	Physical Therapy	66				24
25	Occupational Therapy	67				25
26	Speech Pathology	68				26
27	Electrocardiology	69				27
28	Electroencephalography	70				28
29	Medical Supplies Charged to Patients	71				29
30	Implantable Devices Charged to Patients	72				30
31	Drugs Charged to Patients	73				31
32	Renal Dialysis	74				32
33	ASC (non-distinct part)	75				33
34	Other Ancillary (specify)	76				34
35	Rural Health Clinic (RHC)	88				35
36	Federally Qualified Health Center (FQHC)	89				36
37	Clinic	90				37
38	Emergency Room	91				38
39	Observation Beds	92				39
40	Other Outpatient Service (specify)	93				40
41	TOTAL (sum of lines 8-40)					41

C = Worksheet C line numbers D = Worksheet D-1 line numbers

FORM CMS-2552-10 08-11

COMPUTATION OF ORGAN ACQUISITION COSTS AND CHARGES FOR HOSPITALS WHICH ARE CERTIFIED TRANSPLANT CENTERS	PROVIDER CCN: .... OPO CCN:	PERIOD: FROM.......... TO..........	WORKSHEET D-4, PARTS II

Check applicable box:	[ ] HEART	[ ] LIVER	[ ] PANCREAS	[ ] ISLET
	[ ] KIDNEY	[ ] LUNG	[ ] INTESTINE	[ ] OTHER (specify)

PART II - COMPUTATION OF ORGAN ACQUISITION COSTS (OTHER THAN INPATIENT ROUTINE AND ANCILLARY SERVICE COSTS)

	Computation of the Cost of Inpatient Services of Intems and Residents Not In Approved Teaching Program		Average Cost Per Day (from Wkst. D-2, Part I, col. 4)	Organ Acquisition Days	Organ Acquisition Cost (col. 1 × col. 2)	
		D	1	2	3	
42	Adults & Pediatrics (General routine care)	2				42
43	Intensive Care Unit	3				43
44	Coronary Care Unit	4				44
45	Burn Intensive Care Unit	5				45
46	Surgical Intensive Care Unit	6				46
47	Other Special Care (Specify)	7				47
48	TOTAL (sum of lines 42 through 47)					48

Figure 6.4 Worksheet D-4 Parts I-IV.
Source: http://www.costreportdata.com.

	Computation of the Cost of Outpatient Services of Intems and Residents Not In Approved Teaching Program	Organ Charges (see instructions)		Ratio of Cost to Charges from Wkst. D-2, Part 1, col. 4)	Organ Acquisition Costs (col. 1 × col. 2)	
		1	D	2	3	
49	Rural Health Clinic (RHC)		21			49
50	Federally Qualified Health Center (FQHC)		22			50
51	Clinic		23			51
52	Emergency		24			52
53	Observation Beds		25			53
54	Other Outpatient Service (specify)		26			54
55	TOTAL (sum of lines 49 through 54)					55

D = Worksheet D-2, Part 1, line numbers

08-11 FORM CMS-2552-10

COMPUTATION OF ORGAN ACQUISITION COSTS AND CHARGES FOR HOSPITALS WHICH ARE CERTIFIED TRANSPLANT CENTERS	PROVIDER CCN: .... OPO CCN:	PERIOD: FROM.......... TO..........	WORKSHEET D-4, PARTS III & IV

Check applicable box:	[ ] HEART [ ] KIDNEY	[ ] LIVER [ ] LUNG	[ ] PANCREAS [ ] INTESTINE	[ ] ISLET [ ] OTHER (specify)

PART III - SUMMARY OF COSTS AND CHARGES

		Cost		Charges		
		Part A	Part B	Part A	Part B	
		1	2	3	4	
56	Routine and Ancillary from Part I					56
57	Interns and Residents (inpatient)					57
58	Interns and Residnets (outpatient)					58
59	Direct Organ Acquisition (see instructions)					59
60	Cost of Services of Teaching Physicians (Wkst. D-5, Part II)					60
61	Total (sum of lines 56 thru 60)					61
62	Total Usable Organs (see instructions)					62
63	Medicare Usable Organs (see instructions)					63
64	Ratio of Medicare Usable Organ to Total Usable Organs (line 63 ÷ line 62)					64
65	Medicare Cost/Charges (see instructions)					65
66	Revenue for Organs Sold					66
67	Subtotal (line 65 minus line 66)					67
68	Organs Furnished Part B					68
69	Net Organ Acquisition Cost and Charges (see instructions)					69

PART IV - STATISTICS

		Living Related	Cadaveric	Revenue	
		1	2	3	
70	Organs Excised in Provide R (1)				70
71	Organs Purchased from Other Transplant Hospitals (2)				71
72	Organs Purchased from Non-Transplant Hospitals				72
73	Organs Purchased from OPOs				73
74	Total (sum of lines 70 thru 73)				74
75	Organs Transplanted				75
76	Organs sold to Other Hospitals				76
77	Organs sold to OPOs				77
78	Organs sold to Transplant Hospitals				78
79	Organs sold to Military of VA Hospitals				79
80	Organs sold Outside the U.S.				80
81	Organs sent Outside the U.S. (no revenue received)				81
82	Organs Used for Research				82
83	Unusable/Discarded Organs				83
84	Total (sum of lines 75 through 83 should equal line 74)				84

(1) Organs procured outside your center by a procurement team from your center are not included in the count.

(2) Organs procured outside your center by a procurement team are include in the count.

Figure 6.4 *(Continued)*

acquisition costs are indeed allowable, retaining supporting documentation for pretransplant costs, determining allowable square footage, reconciling transplants performed with financial records, and having a system in place to capture all patient costs that are pretransplant related. This last point is discussed in more depth in the next section.

Flagging of accounts

It is important for transplant centers to capture all the costs associated with pretransplant care of transplant patients since this cost can be reported on the cost report. It involves a well-thought-out process which crosses departmental boundaries with transplant financial staff, hospital billing staff, and reimbursement, all working in cooperation—often referred to "flagging" of accounts or cost report tracking. The process begins when the patient is registered in the patient billing system. The patient is assigned a unique transplant identifier which allows the patient's encounters to be tracked in the billing system. The charges are held until reviewed. The next step is for a transplant staff member, usually a transplant analyst or transplant financial coordinator, to review the charges of each patient who has the identifier and assign their charges as either pretransplant or disease management. It should be noted that it requires a fairly firm grasp of medical terminology and transplant procedures to be able to assign these charges. The charges that are identified as pretransplant are assigned to the cost report. The charges that are identified as disease management are released and billed to the patient's insurance. This process has been further perfected by Henry Ford Transplant Institute, whereby they have created a diagnosis code that allows patient charges to be electronically separated as either pretransplant or disease management by their decision support system. The decision support staff runs a query from a master list of patients and the system accumulates the charges that should be assigned to the cost report, and the results are then manually reviewed for accuracy [12].

Profitability

Transplant program profitability has been an enigma since it has been difficult to fully capture all charges relating to transplant patients, and many patients may also be counted in other service line profit centers such as Cardiology or Gastroenterology. It is a widely held belief among hospital senior leaders that transplant is not profitable. This belief is clearly not valid—transplant as a service line is very profitable for hospitals. Indeed, transplant has been known to provide a "halo effect." This term describes how a service line or program can generate downstream patient encounters and services for a hospital. It is well illustrated in a study by Cohen et al. as to the downstream effect of a hepatology department. Of all hepatology patients, it was liver transplant patients who generated the most hospital revenue for the hepatology department and the hospital overall [13]. This downstream revenue stream is a boon to many hospitals that have struggled with low patient census and profitability.

So, how does one begin the process of determining profitability? First, it requires assistance from finance, decision support, and reimbursement. The ability to flag transplant patient accounts will be required to capture all charges for services and tests. These charges are accumulated, then adjusted for cost with the cost report reimbursement added back in to arrive at the contribution margin. Figure 6.5 shows actual contribution margin for four of the solid organ areas along the continuum of care for a medium-sized transplant program (transplant volume equal to 10 hearts, 10 lungs, 50 livers, and 50 kidneys). Contribution margin is defined as revenue minus the variable cost. The contribution margin for each stage of the continuum of care was determined based on primary and secondary diagnosis codes. In addition, an assumption is that all patients seeking condition management stemmed from the existence of the transplant program. It is interesting to note that in all cases and along the entire continuum of care, the contribution margin is positive. When contribution margin is positive, there is contribution to overhead of the organization. Overhead is defined as the sum of fixed and indirect cost. Fixed cost is typically plant and equipment, and indirect cost is attributable to the nonrevenue-producing areas of the hospital such as housekeeping, dietary, medical records, and administration among others. Figure 6.6 shows the same data with the overhead added, otherwise known as profit margin. Again, the total profit margin for all organ groups is positive. However, there are large differences among the organ groups along the continuum of care. These differences can assist in understanding where along the continuum is the greatest opportunity for cost containment in order to increase profitability.

Heart transplant appears to be the most profitable; however, it is only due to the profitability of the condition management of heart failure patients. Kidney transplant is the second most profitable, with profits coming from pretransplant evaluation and the transplant event. Liver transplant is also quite profitable, with profits generated from the transplant event and condition management. Lung transplant is the least profitable, although profits are generated all along the continuum of care except for the immediate postoperative period. Although this data is unique to one transplant program, it shows the relative profitability of each of the organ groups. Granted, some programs may have higher contribution margins and profitability for some of their organ groups due to implementa-

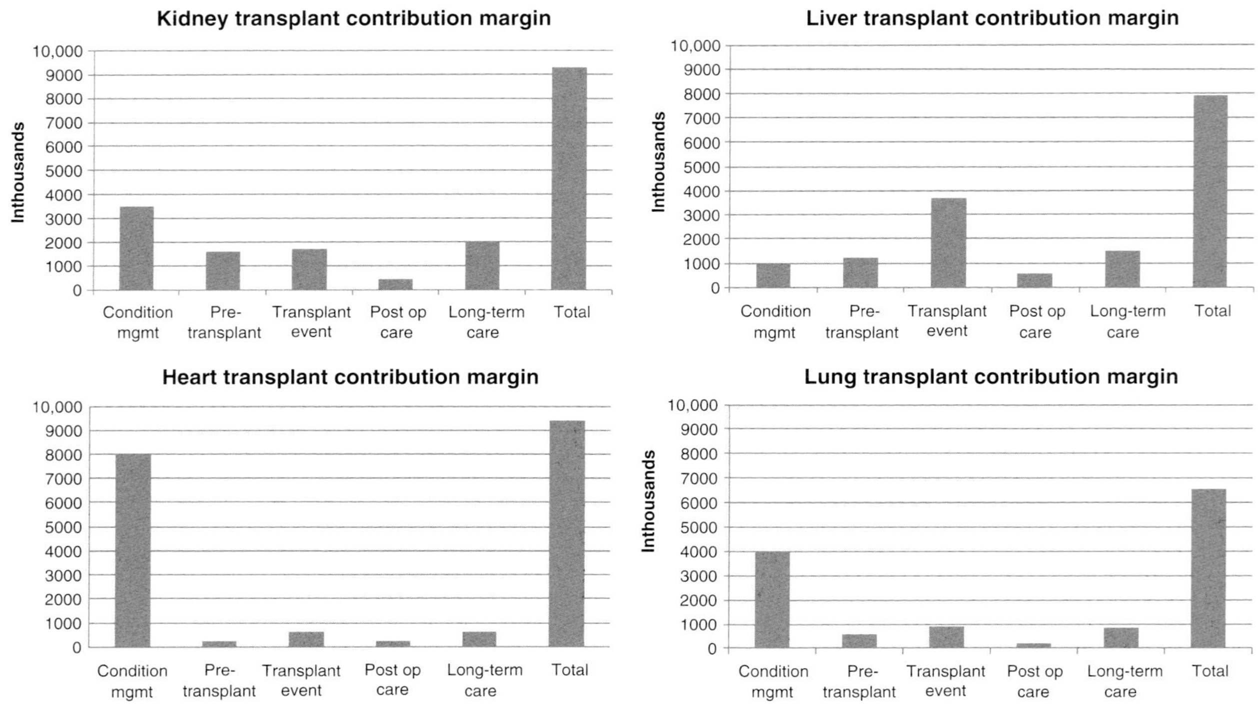

Figure 6.5 Contribution margin for various organs along the continuum of care.

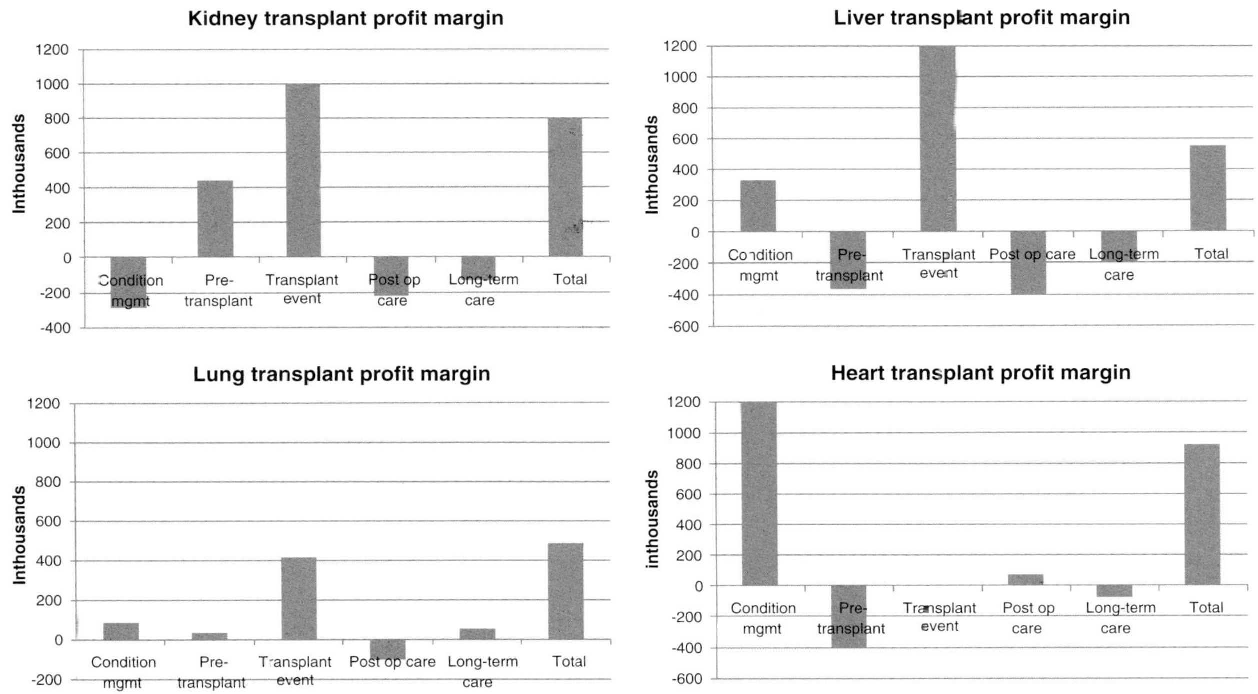

Figure 6.6 Profit margin for various organs along the continuum of care.

tion of cost containment measures, but this data gives a general view of profitability.

Monitoring financial performance

Monitoring financial performance should be an ongoing activity in any transplant program and the responsibility of the transplant administrator or transplant business manager. Similar to overseeing the budget, monitoring financial performance should be a routine activity which includes the development of operating indicators which provide a picture of the financial health of transplant operations. These indicators could include

- Referrals—the number of referrals should be tracked monthly, with referral sources indentified and reviewed at least quarterly. This will indicate if there are changes in referral activity or issues with referring physicians. Referrals are the lifeblood of a transplant program and any decrease in activity should be investigated and acted upon.
- Waitlisted patients—it is important to track the number of patients on the list on a quarterly basis and make note of significant changes. Changes may be due to modifications in listing criteria, problems with the evaluation process, transfers in or out of the program, or changes in MCO networks.
- Number of transplants—since most budgets are based on an estimate of the number of transplants performed per year, any deviation in the number of transplants will impact the financial picture either positively (if more than expected) or negatively (if less than expected). This indicator should be tracked on a monthly basis in order to note any trends, and if the trend continues, an investigation into causes should be instituted. Potential changes in the number of transplants could be due to many factors: changes in the number of waitlisted patients, changes in deceased donor availability, changes in the living donor process, lack of OR capacity, change in turndown rate, etc.
- Cost per case—tracking cost per case should be performed on a quarterly basis and can be obtained from the hospital's finance department. Comparing cost per case by payor to historical averages will give an indication of any major change in utilization or practice.
- Payor mix—the payor mix may also impact financial performance and should be tracked on a quarterly basis. The payor mix may change due to changes in insurance of the patient population, or changes in contracts with MCOs.

Charity care and patient funds

Uncompensated care in the United States is at an all-time high, with more and more Americans finding they can no longer afford the cost of healthcare. According to an American Hospital Association survey of approximately 5000 hospitals, spending on uncompensated care which is charity care and bad debt (or unpaid patient accounts) was 5.9% of total expenses in 2011 [14]. Although this may soon change with the advent of the Patient Protection and Affordable Care Act (Obamacare), many transplant programs will still be affected by patients who cannot afford co-pays, medications, and other necessary items. Patients skip medications and appointments due to economic hardship, which has severe implications for

Transplant Assistance:

HELPHOPELIVE (http://www.helphopelive.org/)
(Formerly NTAF) Helps patients and families facing transplantation or catastrophic injury afford uninsured medically related expenses through grass roots fundraising.

National Foundation for Transplants (NFT) (http://www.transplants.org/)
NTF offers fundraising assistance for organ and tissue transplant patients across the country.

Children's Organ Transplant Association (COTA) (http://www.cota.org/)
COTA helps children, young adults, and people with genetic disorders who need life saving transplants by providing fundraising assistance and family support.

Georgia Transplant Foundation (GTF) (http://gatransplant.org)
GTF is focused on providing both financial and educational assistance during a time that is often overwhelming for those undergoing or waiting for a transplant in the state of Georgia.

National Living Donor Assistance Center (NLDAC) (http://www.livingdonorassistance.org)
Provides assistance for potential living donors who cannot pay for services not covered by insurances such as travel and living expenses.

Pharmacy Assistance:

Partnership for Prescription Assistance (PPA) (http://www.pparx.org/)
PPA helps qualifying patients without prescription coverage get the medications they need through the program that is right for them.

Needy Meds (www.needymeds.org)
Needy Meds helps people find assistance with prescription costs, co pays and premiums, and disease specific expenses.

The HealthWell Foundation (www.healthwellfoundation.org)

Patient Access Network Foundation (www.panfoundation.org)

Figure 6.7 Financial assistance resources for transplant patients.
Source: The Society for Transplant Social Workers (http://www.transplantsocialworker.org/).

transplant center outcomes. In fact, in a survey of US transplant programs, 43% report that more that 10% of their patients are nonadherent due to the ability to pay [15]. It also has implications for transplant staff members who try to find ways to assist these patients, with some even paying for medications out of their own pocket.

Although there are organizations that specialize in assisting transplant patients (Figure 6.7), it is to the benefit of any transplant program to establish a patient assistance fund for patients in need. Many transplant programs do have such a fund and have developed guidelines for fund distribution. Funding for charity care can come from pharmaceutical companies, fund-raising events, and donations.

Please refer to Appendix 8 for further resources.

References

1 Nowicki M. *The Financial Management of Hospitals and Healthcare Organizations*. 4th ed. Chicago: Health Administration Press; 2008:103.
2 Nowicki M. *The Financial Management of Hospitals and Healthcare Organizations*. 4th ed. Chicago: Health Administration Press; 2008:104.
3 Nowicki M. *The Financial Management of Hospitals and Healthcare Organizations*. 4th ed. Chicago: Health Administration Press; 2008:77.
4 Sullivan B. National Trends in Organ Acquisition Costs. 2013. Presentation at the UNOS Transplant Management Forum. New Orleans.
5 Abecasis M. Organ Acquisition Cost Centers Part I: Medicare Regulations-Truth or Consequence. *Am J Transplant*. 2006;6(12):2830–2835.
6 http://www.justice.gov/civil/docs_forms/C-FRAUDS_FCA_Primer.pdf. Accessed October 8, 2013.
7 Beach-Langois M. Transplant cost-report tracking at Henry Ford Transplant Institute and other centers nationwide. *Prog Transplant*. 2011;21(2):172.
8 42CFR 415.70.
9 68CFR 45459.
10 Sullivan B. *National Trends in Organ Acquisition Costs*. 2013. Presentation at the UNOS Transplant Management Forum. New Orleans.
11 Medicare Provider Reimbursement Manual, Form CMS-2552-96 Instructions, http://www.costreportdata.com/instructions/Instr_D60.pdf.
12 Beach-Langois M. Transplant cost-report tracking at Henry Ford Transplant Institute and other centers nationwide. *Prog Transplant*. 2011;21(2):171.
13 Cohen SM. The downstream financial effect of hepatology. *Hepatology*. 2005;41(5): 975.
14 American Hospital Association. Uncompensated Hospital Care Cost Fact Sheet. 2013. http://www.aha.org/content/13/1-2013-uncompensated-care-fs.pdf. Accessed October 8, 2013.
15 Evans RW, Applegate WH, Briscoe DM, et al. Cost-related immunosuppressive medication nonadherence among kidney transplant recipients. *Clin J Am Soc Nephrol*. 2010;5:2325.

CHAPTER 7

Managed Care Contracting

Mindy Scharlin
Transplant and Specialty Services Contracting, Stanford Hospital and Clinics, Stanford, CA, USA

In the age of cost containment and predictability, managed care organizations (MCOs) have the need to develop specialty networks for high-cost services, such as cardiovascular surgery, chronic heart disease, end-stage renal disease, spine surgery, oncology, and transplantation, based on financial and clinical considerations. For the purpose of this chapter, the definition of MCO will include insurance and re-insurance companies (both funded and self-funded health plans) as well as specialty networks, which are not the actual payor of services. Over the last 20 years, MCOs have developed national networks in order to decrease and anticipate costs, expand access to services, and improve the quality of care. By establishing and maintaining a network for tertiary or quaternary services, such as transplantation, MCOs direct business to a limited number of providers, which increases volume and demands lower prices. MCOs usually account for 25–60% of transplant volume for any program (see Table 7.1). This chapter discusses the multifaceted issues of managed care contracting for transplantation services and will include: (i) How does an organization qualify to participate in a transplant network? (ii) How does a transplant program contract and evaluate their profitability with MCOs? and (iii) How does an organization maintain good payor relationships?

Becoming a center of excellence

Many MCOs have established transplant networks, often referred to as "Centers of Excellence" (COE) or "Institutes of Excellence" (IOE). Most transplant programs want this designation in order to access patients. But in order to receive this designation, the transplant program must be certified by CMS, certified by UNOS, and complete a standardized Request for Information (RFI), which is produced by the United Network for Organ Sharing (UNOS). The RFI includes information for the MCO on facilities, quality, volumes, outcomes, staff coverage, and credentials. The template is available on the UNOS Transplant Administrators website at

Transplant Administration, First Edition. Edited by Lisa Norris.

Companion website: www.wiley.com/go/norris/transplantadmin

Table 7.1 Payor mix by organ type

Organ	Percent of transplants paid by Medicare	Percent of transplants paid by private payors
Kidney-living donor	35	59
Kidney-deceased donor	65	27
Kidney/pancreas	52	43
Pancreas alone	16	50
Liver	20	58
Heart	26	54
Lung	33	54

Source: Organ Procurement and Transplantation Network (OPTN) and Scientific Registry of Transplant Recipients (SRTR). OPTN/SRTR 2010 Annual Data Report. Rockville, MD: Department of Health and Human Services, Health Resources and Services Administration, Healthcare Systems Bureau, Division of Transplantation; 2011.

https://portal.unos.org. In addition to the RFI, health plans have additional requirements for qualification that have to be met such as volumes per year and survival statistics.

Almost all MCOs require these RFIs be completed for submission for inclusion in their network, although some MCOs also require each provider to complete a supplement to the UNOS RFI which the MCO will provide. Since the RFI is published once per year, the completed copy should contain all the necessary program information to demonstrate the strength of the program. The process to edit a finalized RFI is difficult, so make sure it is done correctly the first time. Also, the final version should demonstrate why the program should be included in the transplant network, including what makes the program unique and special. Some MCOs review applications for inclusion throughout the year; other MCOs will only review during an annual review cycle, so it is important to know how often new applications are reviewed. An example of the UNOS RFI template can be found in Appendix 9.

Besides completing the standardized RFI and the other credentialing requirements, most MCOs require a site visit. This involves meetings with each organ team, which includes medical and surgical directors, nursing, social work, nutrition, and financial coordinators. In addition to clinical outcomes, most MCOs are also interested in nursing training specific to transplantation services, staff turnover, pharmacist coverage, and clinical coverage for emergencies. The MCO reviews the quality metrics and assesses the facility in its entirety.

Understanding the MCO network and determining the geographic need for adding a transplant program is very important in the business of managed care. Some MCOs have contracted with transplant centers all over the country; others are more selective and limit the number of providers in their network. If there is no transplant center in a particular geographic area, the chances are better in getting a contract. Some transplant networks, albeit few, have a two-tiered transplant network. A two-tiered network is a network with two tiers of providers: the top tier is usually designed as the higher tier where the hospital meets all the contracting guidelines and the second tier, the lower tier, is usually designed for hospitals that do not meet all the contracting guidelines but the network needs that hospital in their network for other business reasons (e.g., no other center located with 500 miles). Often a two-tiered network is driven based on the need of its clients: if they have employees all over the country, the client may insist that a certain provider be included in the network even if it does not meet all the criteria necessary for inclusion in the network. This is usually done to appease the employer group with whom the MCO wants business. The subject of two-tiered networks tends to be quite controversial within the provider community, but the providers have very little control over how the MCOs build their networks. The larger the provider network, the more difficult to get referral volume. In addition, with two-tiered networks, there is usually a benefit difference for the patient: patients who go to the higher tier hospital get a higher benefit, usually a travel benefit which includes airline, lodging, and meals for the patient and one caregiver. Do not rule out the possibility of being included in a network with multitiers since it is a good way to gain access to the network, receive new referrals, and increase volumes.

Before a provider can begin the process of contracting, each program must determine which MCO to approach. The first thing to understand is the transplant program's payor mix—which MCOs are sending business and what percentage of business does each MCO represent? Determine which MCO have the highest volume and address them first. The greater the volume, the more important it is to have a contract with that network. In order to learn more about each MCO and their networks, go to the MCO website and look for information on their specialty networks for transplantation. The next step is to determine the credentialing criteria for each MCO. This is something the managed care department should be able to address as well. Each MCO has minimum volume requirements for each organ type in order to be considered for their network. The volume requirements are different for adult and pediatric programs. An example of criteria for adult volumes (as they represent the majority of transplants in this country) are summarized in Table 7.2. If the program does not meet the guidelines for participation, the transplant program will need to develop a strategy to qualify, which may include addressing programmatic issues that are preventing the program from meeting the MCO guidelines.

Table 7.2 Transplant volume requirements for major payors

Payor	Heart	Lung	Liver	Kidney
Aetna	15/year	20/year	40/year	60/year
Cigna	12/year	12/year	12/year	25/year
Optum	20/year	20/year	35/year (DD) 20/year (LD)	50/year
Humana	10/year	10/year	10/year	10/year

Sources: http://www.aetna.com/healthcare-professionals/documents-forms/Aetna-Institutes-of-Excellence.pdf, https://cignalifesource.com/media/GuidelinesNetworkInclusion_feb.pdf, Optum, personal communication, and https://www.humana.com/provider/support/clinical/transplant/guidelines *(accessed November 1, 2013).*

Once the program meets the MCO's criteria for becoming part of their network, the transplant program, through its managed care department, can begin the process of contract negotiations. All transplant agreements should be structured to maximize reimbursement and profitability of the program. This involves understanding of: (i) the total costs of the program (fixed and variable), (ii) professional costs (if applicable) and whether they will be included or not, (iii) case rates and what they include; and (iv) the level of risk the program is willing to assume.

Understanding internal costs

Understanding the institutional and professional cost structure and the program's total costs is paramount to the success of any transplant program. This is accomplished by having a cost accounting system in the hospital and retrieving cost data on the phases of care for a recent group of cases. The standard acquisition charge should be included to determine the total cost per case (unless carved out). This retrospective review of cases should also surface any outliers. Establishment of the case rate should at least cover the average cost per case (omitting outliers) with the goal of optimizing contribution margin. It is best if the costs can be broken down between fixed and variable, and direct and indirect. The more data available to the managed care department in preparation for the negotiation will help them be successful. It may also be helpful to understand the contracting guidelines of your organization. Are there other guidelines that need to be followed? Is it necessary to cover 100% of total costs or not? What is the profit expectation and is it different for different MCO? If so, what are the differences? Is it based on volume? The answer to these questions will enable the managed care department to meet the goals of the program and the organization (Figure 7.1).

Adjudication: Processing claims according to contract.

Carve Out: A service that is typically part of a case or rate is paid for separately or "carved out." For example, in-patient dialysis would be "carved out" of the case rate for kidney transplantation.

Case Mix: The types of in-patients a hospital or postacute facility treats. The more complex the patient's needs, the greater the amount spent for patient care.

Case-Mix Index: A measure of the relative costliness of treating in an in-patient setting. An index of 1.05 means that the facility's patients are 5% more costly than average.

Case Rate: Flat fee paid for a client's treatment based on their diagnosis and/or presenting problem. For this fee, the provider covers all of the services the client requires for a specific period of time. Also may be called a bundled rate, or flat fee-per-case. Very often used as an intervening step prior to capitation. In this model, the provider is accepting some significant risk, but does have considerable flexibility in how it meets the client's needs. Keys to success in this mode: (1) properly pricing case rate, if provider has control over it and (2) securing a large volume of eligible clients.

Center of Excellence: A network of healthcare providers selected for specific services based on meeting certain criteria or level of quality of care such as outcomes, effectiveness, experience, and cost.

Direct Costs: Those costs comprising direct materials, direct labor, and direct expenses that can be traced directly to specific jobs, products, or services.

Fixed Costs: Costs that do not change with fluctuations in census or in utilization of services.

Global Rate: A case rate that includes both the technical (hospital) and professional reimbursement.

Indirect Costs: Costs that cannot be traced to a particular product. An example is rent or management salaries. They are usually shared by more than one product and are called overhead.

Managed Care Organization: A general term for groups of doctors, hospitals, and other providers that come together in order to enhance the quality and cost-effectiveness of health care. Managed care organizations include health maintenance organizations (HMOs), preferred provider organizations (PPOs), point-of-service plans (POSs), exclusive provider organization (EPOs), etc.

Outlier: A patient whose length of stay or treatment cost differs substantially from the stays or costs of most other patients who received the same service.

Per Diem: A form of payment for services in which the provider is paid a daily fee for specific services or outcomes, regardless of the cost of provision. Per diem rates are paid without regard to actual charges and may vary by level of care, such as medical, surgical, intensive care, skilled care, psychiatric, etc. Per diem rates are usually flat all-inclusive rates.

Variable Cost: A cost of labor, material, or overhead that changes according to the change in the volume of service or production units. Combined with fixed costs, variable costs make up the total cost of service or production. While the total variable cost changes with increased services or production, the total fixed costs stays the same.

Figure 7.1 Managed care basic terms.

Contracting methodologies and reimbursement structure

If the organization does not have contracting guidelines, it is time to develop them. Meet with the finance director and managed care director to begin the conversation on appropriate levels of reimbursement. What is the hospital's overall cost to charge ratio? What is the cost to charge ratio for each organ transplant program? Each organ program may have very different ratios; therefore the organization may determine that the contracting guidelines should be different for each program. Having good data will support the development of appropriate contracting guidelines.

Being familiar with the different contracting methodologies is important since it is through these structures that revenue is delivered to the transplant program(s). A full services transplant agreement usually consists of the following phases of care:

Phases of care—What is included in each phase of care?

Phase I: Evaluation—This phase includes all services necessary to determine whether the patient is a candidate for transplantation. This phase usually includes both institutional and professional services.

Phase II: Pretransplantation—This phase includes all services that are required to keep the patient healthy prior to transplantation. This phase often includes laboratory services and other diagnostics. It would *not* include *non-disease-related services* such as a broken arm or appendicitis.

Phase III: Transplantation—This phase includes all services provided during the in-patient admission. This phase usually begins 24 hours prior to the transplant and continues until discharge.

Phase IV: Post-transplantation—This phase includes institutional and professional services from the day of discharge through a specific period of time (e.g., 60 days). The length of time in this phase is usually determined by how long the program requires the patient to stay close to the hospital before returning home.

Phase V: Follow-up care—This phase includes institutional and professional services from the day after the end of Phase IV for 1 year post transplant.

Based on the phases of care listed above, the reimbursement structure can include a combination of the following but only one methodology is used per phase of care:

Phase I: Evaluation

- Percent of charges
- Per diem (for in-patient only)
- Case rate (not too common)

Phase II: Pretransplantation
- Percent of charges
- Per diem (in-patient only)

Phase III: Transplantation
- Case rate with stop loss
- Case rate without stop loss
- Per diem with stop loss
- Per diem without stop loss

Phase IV: Post-transplantation
- Included in Phase III reimbursement
- Per diem
- Percent of charges

Phase V. Follow-up care
- Percent of charges
- Per diem (in-patient only)

It is important to note that if the facility has a general services agreement with the MCO, then usually Phase I, Phase II, and Phase V are paid under the general services agreement; only Phase III and Phase IV are paid under the transplant agreement under the COE or IOE network.

Reimbursement can be structured in many different ways. Within a case rate methodology, reimbursement for institutional services can be included with reimbursement for professional services. This is called "global" rate. Reimbursement can also be separate by entity; in other words, there can be a case rate for the institutional services and a separate case rate for professional services. In both of these reimbursement structures, the invoices for services should be batched as a package and submitted to the MCO along with a cover sheet that indicates the expected reimbursement due. This is the best way to assure payment will be correct. (See Appendix 10.) Global rates and case rates are most commonly associated with Phase III (Transplantation). Case rates are sometimes negotiated for Phase I (Evaluation), but is not that common or recommended because (i) usually no stop loss protection is included and (ii) if the hospital accepts tests results from other providers for the evaluation phase of care, it makes no sense to have a case rate for services the hospital does not provide.

Carved-out services

During the transplant admission, all services are included in the case rate unless they have been "carved-out" from the case rate. Services that tend to be "carved out" are generally services that are very costly, services that do not occur in the majority of cases, or services that the hospital does not provide. A list of these typical services is provided in Table 7.3 and often includes ventricular assist devices (VADs), high-cost pharmaceuticals,

Table 7.3 Transplant carve-out services

Transportation
Prescription and non-prescription agents
In-patient dialysis
Dental services
Home health
Rehabilitation services—in-patient and outpatient
Chemotherapy and radiation
Plasmapheresis
Housing
Organ procurement
Telemedicine
Assist devices
High-dollar blood products
Services provided by another provider

and organ acquisition (including the cost of transportation for the organ). Specifically, in the area of heart transplantation, technology is growing rapidly. Not only are patients able to be kept alive on a VAD until an appropriate organ is available, but in addition to what is referred to as a "bridge-to-transplant," some patients now can have a VAD for the rest of their life, termed "destination therapy." Be aware that even though destination therapy is cutting edge, the device and supportive equipment are very costly. Many hospitals have found that including these devices—and their supporting equipment, such as battery packs and other supplies and materials—is too costly to include in the case rate. Therefore, many hospitals have found that by carving these devices out of the case rate, they can still collect the cost of providing the device (at 100% of invoice cost) and keep the case rate at an appropriate level. These types of advancements and changes in technology have to be communicated to the managed care department so they can contract for these services appropriately.

In addition, more and more MCOs are asking hospitals to carve out high-cost pharmaceuticals. This is because the MCOs know that the hospital's mark up on drugs is extremely high, often much more than 200% of the cost, which will trigger the contract's stop loss. Before agreeing to a drug carve out, the hospital has to know the cost and charge of the drugs and what percentage of the case rate is allocated to pharmaceuticals. Since pharmacy pricing can be very complicated, the managed care department should work with the pharmacy department to learn about the cost and charge structure in order to evaluate whether carving out any drugs can be accomplished. Sometimes the high-cost drugs are posted to one revenue center so they are fairly simple to identify. If not, carving this out will be a very manual process, and since the cost of the drugs is so high (and not controlled by the hospital) and are used in all transplant cases, MCOs most likely will be demanding this carve out more and more in the future, and it is very possible that by doing so, it will be disadvantageous to the hospital.

Another service that is sometimes carved out of the case rate is the organ and its related transportation cost. Charges for the organ and its transportation are billed directly to the hospital by the local organ procurement organization (OPO). The costs of organs—and the transportation getting from the donor hospital to the recipient hospital—vary by region. The OPOs are independent organizations and are structured and run separately from each other; so not all OPOs bill the same amounts. What is consistent between all the OPOs is that the cost of an organ is quite high. What is not consistent is how the OPOs charge for the organs and for transporting the organs from outside their service area. OPOs will invoice additional charges when they procure an organ from outside their service area. Unfortunately, the hospital does not have a way to bill the MCO for this additional cost, resulting in the hospital bearing this financial burden. Depending on how many organs the hospital receives from out of area, this could have a substantial financial impact on the transplant program. Many hospitals these days are getting organs from outside of their region due to the allocation guidelines; so the cost of transportation may be a significant cost that could be passed on to the hospital. In terms of reimbursement, if an item is carved out and paid separately from the case rate, then it should *not* be included in the stop loss or outlier calculation. This should be made clear in the contract and should be communicated to the business office and finance department as well.

The art of stop loss

How the reimbursement is structured has a huge impact on the transplant program's profitability. Case rates are only part of the reimbursement methodology. Every contract should include some type of stop loss, which helps protect the hospital from outlier cases. If patients have a long length of stay (LOS) or a complication, stop loss provides additional reimbursement to cover those costs. In the ideal world, stop loss cases should only comprise about 20% of all the cases. But in the current market, stop loss cases make up much more than 20%. The reason for this is that the case rates negotiated by MCOs are market driven. If the case rates are too high, the MCO cannot sell their network to their clients. Therefore, case rates are set too low for hospitals to cover their costs without collecting additional compensation through a stop loss methodology.

There are several different types of stop losses. Hospitals vary in their preferred stop loss methodology. Some factors that may influence a hospital's preference are based on case mix and LOS variances. The higher the case mix, the less ability the hospital can project charges or LOS. For example, a program that just performs kidney transplants has a much better idea of their case mix, but a program that performs heart or liver transplants has a much wider variety of cases and most likely a higher case mix index. There are also geographic differences in contracting methodologies, as well. In some parts of the country, transplant reimbursement is based on diagnosis-related group (DRG) reimbursement, and therefore no stop loss is expected or negotiated. In other parts of the country, DRG reimbursement for commercial plans is unheard of. When deciding what works best for the facility, reliable data on cost and LOS must be available. Without data, the negotiator cannot negotiate from a position of strength and knowledge. The other main role that stop loss plays is sharing financial risk with the MCO. Financial risk should not be the burden of only the provider; it should be shared between the hospital and the MCO. As you will see the following examples, stop loss based on charges nets a higher reimbursement. Even though MCOs may complain they are at a hospital's mercy if they are paying based on charges, at least charges reflect the amount of services that are being delivered. Stop loss that is based on the number of days a patient remains in the hospital may not net the hospital a level of reimbursement that covers 100% of the hospital's cost of delivering care.

The following are examples of stop loss methodologies. The attachment point is the trigger point where additional payment can be made. Each example shows the calculated payment as well as the percentage of charges covered in each scenario.

First Dollar: If total billed charges are greater than the attachment point, payment equals the percent reimbursement multiplied by the total billed charges *in lieu of* the transplant case rate.

1 "First Dollar" Stop Loss Example

Transplant case rate	$100,000
Stop loss attachment point	$200,000
Percent reimbursement	60%
Total billed charges	$350,000

Calculation:

Total payment : $350,000 × 60% = $210,000 (charges coverage = 60%)

Second Dollar: If total billed charges are greater than the attachment point, payment shall be the case rate plus percentage above the attachment point.

2 "Second Dollar" Stop Loss Example

Transplant case rate	$100,000
Stop loss attachment point	$200,000
Percentage above stop loss	60%
Total billed charges	$350,000

Calculation:

Total payment = (Total billed charges – stop loss) × percentage + case rate

$350,000 – $200,000 = $150,000 × 60% = $90,000 + $100,000

Total payment = $190,000 (charges coverage = 54%)

Per diem outlier: If in-patient LOS is greater than the allowed LOS, payment shall be the case rate plus number of days greater than the allowed LOS multiplied by the negotiated per diem.

3 "Per Diem Outlier" Example

Transplant case rate	$100,000
Total billed charges	$350,000
Allowed LOS	20 days
Outlier per diem	$3000

Calculation:

LOS on this admission: 30 days

10 days @$3000: $30,000

Case rate: $100,000

Total payment: $130,000 (charges coverage = 37%)

Floor outlier: Case rate will be paid for the entire admission but hospital shall never receive less than the floor.

4 "Floor Outlier"

Transplant case rates	$100,000
Floor	50%
Total billed charges	$350,000

Calculation:

Case rate: $100,000

Floor calculation: $350,000 × 50% = $175,000

Total payment: $175,000 (charges coverage = 50%)

An example of 2011 average charges in the United States, by organ type, is shown in Table 7.4. This table offers data on both institutional and

Table 7.4 2011 estimated billed charges per transplant (in dollars)

Transplant	30 days pretransplantation	Procurement	Transplant event	Physician—transplant event	180 days post-op
Kidney	17,000	67,200	91,200	18,500	50,800
Liver	25,400	71,000	316,900	46,600	93,900
Pancreas	17,000	65,000	108,900	17,800	61,400
Kidney/pancreas	20,800	102,500	194,900	34,700	100,400
Heart	47,200	80,400	634,300	67,700	137,800
Single lung	10,300	73,100	302,900	33,500	117,700
Double lung	21,400	90,300	458,500	56,300	142,600
Heart/lung	56,800	130,500	777,700	81,000	169,100
Intestine	55,100	78,500	787,900	104,100	146,600

Source: Data from Milliman. *U.S. Organ and Tissue Transplant Cost Estimates and Discussion*. April 2011. p. 4.

professional charges for the most of the transplant care as well as charge date for the organ acquisition. Since there is wide range of charges for providing the care as well as what institutions charge for the organ acquisition, this document should be used as a benchmark only.

Contract renewal

Contracts are negotiated either with an automatic renewal or with a hard end date. There are advantages and disadvantages to both types. When a contract is first negotiated, usually a 1- or 2-year initial term is negotiated. That means that the contract cannot be terminated within this initial period. This gives both parties a chance to refer business and see if the contract is worthwhile and successful. From the MCO perspective, it is good for the MCO to maintain their network without too much fluctuation of providers. Imagine if a MCO's network changed from year to year—that would provide for a lot of instability for the MCO when trying to sell their products to potential clients! The advantage to the hospital for signing a multiyear agreement is to see how much referral business can be obtained in the near term. It usually takes at least a year or two to begin to see new volume coming to the hospital. If the contract is with a MCO that is well known in the market with established clients, an automatic renewal may be a good idea. This way the hospital does not have to renegotiate the terms every year. If the hospital agreed to very competitive rates in order to get into the network, a hard term date may be best, then after the initial term of the agreement, the hospital can re-evaluate the contract to ensure the hospital is not losing money. How much new volume came to the hospital? How did the contract perform? Were there any significant issues between the parties? Were claims paid correctly and timely according to the contract terms? A hard term creates a deadline that compels the hospital to evaluate the agreement; if the contract is not renegotiated, there is no contract. Also, depending on if the hospital has an annual automatic charge master increase, and depending on the structure of the agreement, a contract that is "evergreen" or one that automatically renews each year could be beneficial to the hospital. In addition, if the contract has dollar-based stop loss, one that is triggered by charges, there may be no advantage to renegotiating the terms of the contract on an annual basis. For example, if the hospital's charges increase 5% per year, the overall charges per case will increase 5% that year; therefore, stop loss will be reached earlier and revenue will automatically be increased by 5%. Last, if the contract is not profitable, it is perfectly acceptable to walk away. An example of a contract can be found in Appendix 11.

Collaboration with the business office

When the managed care department staff is developing and negotiating a contract methodology, the business office staff should be consulted early on in the process to make sure the structure and reimbursement methodology can be correctly adjudicated. It is important that the business office can administer whichever reimbursement structure is in the contract. If the staff cannot batch and package the bills by entity—institutional and professional—or by phase of care, this will present a problem. The reimbursement structure may require manual adjudication, although this is very common in transplant billing departments. An example of a standard rate exhibit is included in Appendix 11.

The most efficient business office is one where there is dedicated staff for transplant claim adjudication. Consistency translates to efficiency. Having the same people working these claims all the time will be very beneficial. If the managed care department negotiates a methodology that the business office cannot execute, it could be a minor disaster, since there is no ability to collect the agreed-upon monies owed. The two departments should work together closely, with the support of the administration, to ensure that billing and reimbursement are performed efficiently.

Fostering a good working relationship between the managed care department and the business office is key. Both departments should have regular meetings (e.g., quarterly) so that communication channels can stay open. The managed care department can report to the business office any issues with the contracts, problems with a negotiation, or changes with the

MCO, particularly the MCO's Operations Manual. It also gives the business office the opportunity to share problems they are having with individual MCO, either with denials, incorrect or late payments, or other operational issues. It can be helpful for the transplant administrator to occasionally participate in these meetings to become aware of any significant issues that may affect patients.

Operationalizing a contract

What goes in to operationalizing a contract? Once the contract has been fully executed, all the appropriate departments have to be notified. Typically, the following departments need to know about any completed contracts:

- Hospital business office or patient financial services
- Professional billing office(s)
- Admitting
- Financial counseling
- Utilization review
- Transplant administration
- Managed care
- Ancillary departments, such as home pharmacy, home infusion

See Figure 7.2 for an example of the information flow between the various departments.

It is beneficial to hold regular meetings with representatives of these departments to make sure they are up-to-date on new contracts, changes to existing contracts, and how to implement such changes. Each department will want to know how the changes affect their department especially if the contract dictates new processes or requirements. If a tool does not already exist, a matrix should be developed by the managed care department that indicates all the contracts, and which services are included or excluded from the phases of care and from the contract overall.

When meeting with the many departments that are affected by the terms of any agreement, it is important to emphasize that when specific MCO issues do arise, each department should track the specific MCO concerns. At the end of the contract year, when it is time to renegotiate the contract terms, each department should submit their issues, such as timely payment, accurate payment, authorization problems, and concurrent review—anything that has been a regular problem to the managed care department. This information will help during the renegotiation process and will provide information to the managed care department that can be communicated to the MCO if specific terms need to be changed.

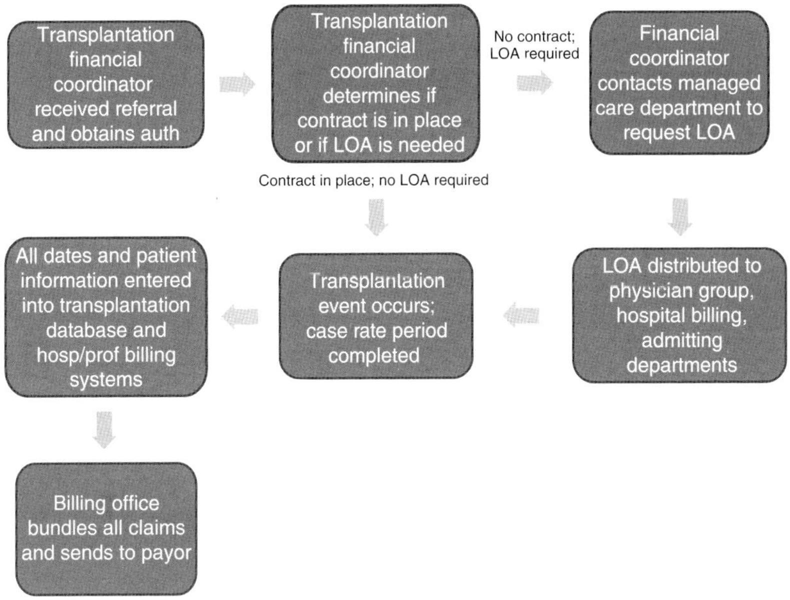

Figure 7.2 Transplant contract information flow.

Some services may not be provided at the facility and are subcontracted out to another facility. Services such as outpatient pharmacy, home pharmacy, home infusion, and rehabilitation are services often subcontracted out. Are these services included or excluded from the agreement? If they are included, who has the financial risk for these services if they are provided at the transplant facility versus provided by a subcontracted facility? It should be very clear if the hospital has risk for services that are provided *outside* of the transplant facility. Are there billing systems in place for this to take place? Is an agreement in place between the facility and the subcontractor that makes reimbursement and payment timing clear? If the hospital has financial risk for any subcontracted service, make sure there is an internal system put in place to refer, authorize, and agree on payment terms before sending a patient to a subcontractor.

Contract performance

Contract performance review and evaluation is critical to the financial viability of a program and ultimately to the hospital. Contract review should be performed at minimum on an annual basis to assess contract performance and find problems as early as possible. Contract performance can be assessed more often if billing and payment issues are problematic. The hospital should have a good cost accounting system to assist in this process. Usually, data are provided by the managed care department or the finance department. Data should include all commercial MCO volumes, LOS, total charges, total costs, and any other financial terms that are part of the agreement. The managed care department usually leads these meetings and includes the transplant administrator, the medical and surgical transplant directors, and business office representatives from both hospital and physician group. This is a good way to assess payment errors, discuss outlier cases, and share program information that could affect the data (e.g., changes in protocol, unusual circumstances in a particular case, capacity issues, etc.). This type of data review helps address whether the contract was successful and what should be done in the coming year to make changes, if necessary. Meetings that occur regularly will help to address issues early in the process. These types of meetings may also help address issues before they are billed to the MCO as well as issues such as payment turnaround time. The earlier the problems are identified, the earlier they will be resolved which ensures hospital success. Also, the program should ask when was the last time a case by case analysis of costs per case was prepared. This type of exercise will influence profitability of the program and make it more competitive in the marketplace.

Benefit levels

Over the last several years, a significant area of concern for transplant providers is the level of benefit coverage patients have through their health plans. Several states have begun to require commercial MCOs to cover a minimum level of transplant benefits. Unfortunately, the minimum benefit has been misconstrued and has become the *maximum benefit*. For example, if a state mandates that every commercial plan has to cover a minimum of $250,000 for transplantation services for a patient's lifetime, the health plan has implemented coverage with a *maximum transplant bene*fit of $250,000. Hence, it is extremely important that each transplant program has criteria in place regarding necessary benefit coverage before establishing a relationship with the patient. Each transplant program's financial coordinators must know what the program's criteria for minimum benefit levels before accepting a referral. They must know the hospital's process if a patient does not have enough coverage at the time of referral. A financial assessment tool should be developed if the program does not already have one in place. This tool should be reviewed every year or two to make sure the criteria are still applicable. See Appendix 12. It is perfectly acceptable for different organ programs in the same hospital to have different benefit minimums since the average charges for each program are most likely different from one and other.

Relationship with MCOs

Finally, developing and maintaining good working relationships with the MCO is paramount to having a successful relationship. As issues come up throughout the year, it makes it easier to resolve issues when there is a good working relationship between all parties. During a MCO site visit, which is a contractual obligation of most contracts, it is a good time for the program's clinical staff to meet the MCO's clinical staff in order to meet face-to-face and form a good relationship. Agreeing to ways of communicating at this time will help build and maintain good working relationships between clinical staff from the hospital and MCO. Exchanging contact numbers and discussing expectations for communication is very useful in building a new relationship. Some transplant physicians are now providing their cell phone number to the MCO medical director so patient referral and clinical issues can be discussed immediately, 24/7. This is one way to make the leadership of the program easily accessible to the MCO, and it conveys to the MCO that the program is serious about maintaining an excellent working relationship.

Throughout the year, as the transplant program updates any marketing materials, it is a good idea to send them to the MCO contacts: the medical director, contract manager, and the transplant case managers. If clinical issues come up during the year, make it a point to resolve them as quickly as possible; pick up the telephone and call the person at the MCO to let them know the issue is being addressed. Encourage the transplant program leadership to make themselves available to the MCO in ways that the MCO knows the transplant staff is responsive to all their issues and concerns.

Remember: the MCO is your client. They send you business and maintaining good relationships will encourage them to send you more! Be honest and direct in your communication: if you do not know the answer to the inquiry, let them know their question will be investigated and a response will be forthcoming as soon as possible. Good relationships are the key to success!

Please refer to Appendices 9–12 for further resources.

CHAPTER 8

Quality Assessment and Performance Improvement

Lisa Norris
Transplant Leadership Institute LLC, San Antonio, TX, USA

Quality and Performance Improvement has become a topic of upmost importance to healthcare organizations, regulators, insurers, providers, and patients. Evidence of this can found in the push for evidence-based medicine, pay for performance, patient safety goals, and accountable care organizations. This trend has also been felt in the transplant community. Transplant is already one of the most transparent areas of medicine, one where the public can access detailed information about every center and every organ system treated in that transplant program. This transparency is even further illuminated in the quest for quality and quality assurance. CMS mandates the establishment of a quality program for any transplant center seeking participation in their programs. The exact regulatory language is:

> "Transplant centers must develop, implement and maintain a written comprehensive, data-driven QAPI program designed to monitor and evaluate performance of all transplantation services, including services provided under contract or arrangement" (CFR 482.96).

However, most importantly, a quality program should be developed to ensure program effectiveness and clinical excellence. High-performing transplant centers have found ways to incorporate three key practices to improve the quality of care:

- Use patient care protocols to guide and standardize patient care.
- Continuously improve clinical care.
- Cultivate a culture of quality and performance improvement.

The HRSA Transplant Center Growth and Management Collaborative Best Practices Final Report found that standardized patient care protocols were key drivers to high performance. Protocols or guidelines provide a mechanism for coordinated team action for providing clinical care. These protocols also allow providers to increase efficiency, ensure safety, and

Transplant Administration, First Edition. Edited by Lisa Norris.

Companion website: www.wiley.com/go/norris/transplantadmin

improve patient outcomes [1]. Patient protocols should be developed for pre-, post- and in-patient care—it is widely known that in-patient clinical pathways have dramatically decreased the length of stay, thereby improving the cost of care and margin. Protocols should be reviewed at least annually to allow for advances in care.

Having protocols in place is a good start. Next, there should be a program where the team strives to continuously improve care based on protocol compliance, data collection, and comparing outcomes to benchmarks. In order to formalize this approach, the transplant program must develop its own well-defined structure that interfaces with the organization's overall quality program. A Quality Assurance and Performance Improvement (QAPI) committee should be established, whose members are influential in ensuring quality within the transplant program. Members, at a minimum, should include transplant surgeons, transplant physicians, transplant administrator, transplant coordinators, transplant social worker, transplant dietician, transplant pharmacist, OPO representative, living donor advocate, and transplant floor nurses. This committee should meet regularly and at a minimum quarterly. A member of this committee should sit on the hospital's quality committee.

The QAPI program plan should also be defined and described in the transplant program's policy and procedure manual and should include the following elements:

- Overall plan description
- Organizational structure/chart which shows how the transplant quality committee reports up through the overall hospital quality program
- Purpose, goals, and objectives of the QAPI program
- Description of the QAPI committee
- Roles and responsibilities of committee members (see Table 8.1)
- Mechanisms of reporting, i.e., minutes and distribution
- Reporting and initiatives relating to adverse events
- Criteria to be used for quality assessment
- Methods used to collect and analyze data

Table 8.1 QAPI Committee responsibilities

- Determine annual QAPI measures
- Prioritize QAPI measures
- Evaluate QAPI measures against benchmarks
- Assess progress and effectiveness of improvement projects
- Identify further needed action or resources
- Review status of performance improvement projects
- Review all adverse events and participate in root-cause analyses
- Document all meetings
- Report regularly to overall organizational quality committee

- Methodology to be used for performance improvement activities (discussed later in this chapter)
- Frequency of meetings [2]

Quality assessment

First, a good-quality program should have mechanisms to assess quality. The definition of quality assessment is the measurement of quality. This would include establishing objective criteria to be evaluated, measuring these criteria, and comparing these criteria with benchmarks or standards. CMS regulations in CFR 482.96 state:

> "The transplant center's QAPI program must use objective measures to evaluate the center's performance with regard to transplantation activities and outcomes."

Usually, these criteria or measures relate to transplant processes or patient outcomes across the three phases of transplant care: pretransplant, in-patient, and post-transplant. Transplant programs may select any number of criteria; however, CMS regulations require that the criteria be applied to each phase of care for both donors and recipients. Examples of criteria are found in Table 8.2. Please note that the criteria in Table 8.2 are very specific and measurable. Once the criteria have been established for the program, benchmarks should be selected. These benchmarks are a point of reference or a standard and can be any of the following: best practices, regulatory data, national benchmarks, the program's own established targets, variances in care, or patient outcomes. Use of benchmarks

Table 8.2 Examples of criteria

Number of transplants
Patient survival 1 year
Graft survival 1 year
Rejection episodes
Number of infections
Reoperations
Number of complications
Readmissions within 30 days post-transplant
Length of stay
Number of referrals per month
Average days from referral to listing
ABO verification at time of surgery
Notification of removal from the waitlist within 10 business days
Cold ischemia time
Number of declined organs
Mortality on the waitlist

and comparing a program against the best is necessary for a program to attain clinical excellence and to have continuous improvement. For those transplant centers who are members of the University Health System Consortium (UHC), transplant-specific data (based on diagnostic-related group or DRG) are available from other member organizations for comparison. Still applicable, although dated, is the UHC benchmarking project field book for transplant services published in 2004 [3]. This booklet is still one of the best benchmarking studies to date for liver and kidney transplantation. Data from that study are available in Figure 8.1. Other national benchmarks may be found in articles on various websites, particularly the Agency for Healthcare Research and Quality website (ahrq.gov) and the International Society for Heart and Lung Transplantation website under guidelines at www.ishlt.org.

After deciding the criteria to be measured and the benchmarks to compare against, a transplant program should develop a method to collect the necessary data. Data collection and reporting can be much easier if a transplant database or electronic medical record is employed; however, data can be mined from manual methods such as chart review, audits, mock surveys, and observations. Data should then be collected or aggregated and analyzed. Data analysis can take many different forms. The simplest methodology is determining the mean and median for the set of data and comparing it to previous data sets and benchmarks. This data is usually collected over a specific timeframe and is presented in the form of a chart, scorecard, dashboard, or others. An example of a dashboard can be found in Figure 8.2. Regulations do not stipulate which tools to use but state that some form of useful tool is employed by the program. Statistical analysis and significance may or may not be necessary. Once the data are analyzed and compiled, it is reported to the QAPI committee so that they can discuss the data. Key questions of committee members should be: (i) is the data valid? (ii) should more data be collected? (iii) are there trends in the data? (iv) or is this an opportunity for performance improvement?

Performance improvement

Once a data-driven quality assessment program has been established, performance improvement activities should be considered for those areas where the program falls short of benchmarks. Generally speaking, performance improvement is defined as measuring or evaluating a particular process and then revising the process to close the gap between actual and expected performance. CMS regulations state:

> "The transplant center must take actions that result in performance improvements and track performance to ensure that improvements are sustained" (CFR 482.96).

Appendix A

Appendix A

Improvement and Effectiveness Performance Opportunity Summary - Kidney

Transplant Services Benchmarking Project 2003

This document provides a comparison of your organization's performance to other participants. **The information is intended to create internal discussion about improvement possibilities.** Please note that performance measures do not consider all operating differences. This report reflects your organization's performance for key measures in the areas of clinical effectiveness and operational efficiency for transplant services. Improvement opportunities should be evaluated if there is a checked box or a quantified value shown under the "Performance Opportunity" column. Quantified opportunities are for a year. Detailed supporting information is available in the aggregate clinical reports and the operational survey reports on the UHC Web site at www.uhc.edu (select "Improvement & Effectiveness", "Benchmarking", and "Transplant Services"). For more information about the UHC Transplant Services Benchmarking Project, contact the project leaders: Danielle Carrier at 630/954-3794 or carrier@uhc.edu or Jackie Dostal at 630/645-8160 or dostal@uhc.edu.

Performance Measures	Best Decile	Best Quartile	Benchmark	Potential Performance Opportunity if Best Quartile Performance Achieved
1. Prophylactic antibiotic given 30 minutes prior to incision	43.3%	30.3%	75%	
2. Cold ischemic time (deceased donors only/hours)	12.1	14.9	14.9	
3. Operating room time (patient in room to patient out /median hours)	3.5	3.7	3.7	
4. CMV[1]prophylaxis for patient at risk	100.0%	100.0%	100.0%	
5. Units of red blood cells per patient administered within 48 hours after incision (units/all patients)	0.0	0.1	0.1	
6. Reoperations during initial hospital stay (excludes retransplants and biopsy)	0.0%	0.8%	0.8%	
7. Post-transplant ICU utilization	3.3%	10.0%	10.0%	
8. Infection rate	0.0%	3.3%	3.3%	
9. Post-transplant dialysis of patients receiving organs from deceased donors	5.6%	12.5%	12.5%	
10. Postprocedure LOS (median days)	4.0	5.0	5.0	
11. LOS O/E	0.8	0.9	1.0	
12. Cost O/E	0.8	0.9	1.0	
13. Program FTEs per 1,000 outpatient visits	2.3	3.2	3.2	
14. Salary cost per 1,000 outpatient visits	$82,444	$125,534	$125,534	
15. Readmission rate within 90 days	15.8%	21.9%	21.9%	
16. Graft survival rate at 1 year	94.6%	92.8%	92.8%	

Source:
- Clinical data collection of up to 30 kidney and 30 liver transplants between 10/01/02 and 3/31/03
- Operational survey for 12-month period ending 12/31/02 for heart, lung, liver, kidney, pancreas, and kidney/pancreas transplants
- Clinical Data Base (CDB) same organs and time frame as the operational survey

[1]CMV: Prophylaxis antiviral drugs received by seropositive recipients on induction therapy or R-/D+

- printed June 1, 2004 -

28 UHC Transplant Services 2003 Benchmarking Project Field Book

Figure 8.1 University HealthSystem Consortium Transplant Benchmarking Summaries for Liver and Kidney

These areas of underperformance should also be prioritized in order of importance for the program—it may be financial, clinical, or regulatory. Usually, a smaller subset of the QAPI committee, along with specially selected staff, undertakes these performance improvement initiatives by selecting one of the many methodologies for process improvement. One of the most well-known and applicable methodologies for transplant programs is Plan-Do-Study-Act.

Improvement and Effectiveness Performance Opportunity Summary - Liver
Transplant Services Benchmarking Project 2003

This document provides a comparison of your organization's performance to other participants. **The information is intended to create internal discussion about improvement possibilities.** Please note that performance measures do not consider all operating differences. This report reflects your organization's performance for key measures in the areas of clinical effectiveness and operational efficiency for transplant services. Improvement opportunities should be evaluated if there is a checked box or a quantified value shown under the "Performance Opportunity" column. Quantified opportunities are for a year. Detailed supporting information is available in the aggregate clinical reports and the operational survey reports on the UHC Web site at www.uhc.edu (select "Improvement & Effectiveness", "Benchmarking", and "Transplant Services"). For more information about the UHC Transplant Services Benchmarking Project, contact the project leaders: Danielle Carrier at 630/954-3794 or carrier@uhc.edu or Jackie Dostal at 630/645-8160 or dostal@uhc.edu.

Performance Measures	Best Decile	Best Quartile	Benchmark	Potential Performance Opportunity if Best Quartile Performance Achieved
1. Prophylactic antibiotic given 30 minutes prior to incision	27.3%	20.0%	75%	
2. Cold ischemic time (deceased donors only/hours)	5.3	6.1	6.1	
3. Operating room time (patient in room to patient out /median hours)	6.5	7.4	7.4	
4. CMV[1]prophylaxis for patient at risk	100.0%	100.0%	100.0%	
5. Units of red blood cells per patient administered within 48 hours after incision (units/all patients)	3.5	6.0	6.0	
6. Reoperations during initial hospital stay (excludes retransplants and biopsy)	4.3%	6.7%	6.7%	
7. Infection rate	6.7%	11.4%	11.4%	
8. Post-transplant dialysis of patients receiving organs from deceased donors	0.0%	3.5%	3.5%	
9. Postprocedure LOS (median days)	7.0	8.0	8.0	
10. LOS O/E	0.8	0.9	1.0	
11. Cost O/E	0.8	0.8	1.0	
12. Program FTEs per 1,000 outpatient visits	2.8	4.4	4.4	
13. Salary cost per 1,000 outpatient visits	$127,305	$163,653	$163,653	
14. Readmission rate within 90 days	23.4%	33.8%	33.8%	
15. Graft survival rate at 1 year	85.9%	84.5%	84.5%	

Source:
- Clinical data collection of up to 30 kidney and 30 liver transplants between 10/01/02 and 3/31/03
- Operational survey for 12-month period ending 12/31/02 for heart, lung, liver, kidney, pancreas, and kidney/pancreas transplants
- Clinical Data Base (CDB) same organs and time frame as the operational survey

[1]CMV: Prophylaxis antiviral drugs received by seropositive recipients on induction therapy or R-/D+

- printed June 1, 2004 -

UHC Transplant Services 2003 Benchmarking Project Field Book 29

Figure 8.1 (*Continued*) *Source*: University HealthSystem Consortium. 2004. Transplant Services. 2003 Benchmarking Project Field Book. reproduced with permission.

Plan-Do-Study-Act

Plan-Do-Study-Act or PDSA was introduced in the 1930s and was modified by the renowned quality authority, W. Edwards Deming. The cycle provides a framework for developing and testing ideas which will lead to performance or process improvement. The steps to PDSA are the following:

Plan: State the objectives; determine the needed improvements; design a process change; define the who, what, when, and where; identify what data to collect in order to determine whether the desired outcome has been achieved.

Metric	Benchmark Source	Benchmark	Q1 FY11	Q2 FY11	Q3 FY11	Q4 FY11
LOS	UHC	5.0 Days	10.0 days	7.0 days	9.5	8.0
Readmission with 90 days	UHC	21.9%	63.7%	27.3%	66.3%	25.0%
Cold time	UHC	14.54 hours	18.2 hours	17.0 hours	20.0 hours	25.0 hours
OR time	Internal standard	4.5 hours	5.0 hours	4.42 hours	4.23 hours	5.1 hours
Rejection rate	Internal standard	<20%	16%	10%	8%	10%
Delayed graft function	Internal standard	<20%	6%	3%	10%	13%
Lymphocele	Internal standard	<10%	1.2%	0%	0%	0%
ABO verification prior to listing	Internal standard	100%	100%	99%	100%	100%
Removal from waitlist within 24 hours of transplantation	Internal standard	100%	89%	88%	95%	100%
Completion of surgical consent	Internal standard	100%	100%	100%	100%	100%
Compliance with multiple listing policy	Internal standard	100%	80%	80%	95%	100%
Forms submission to UNOS (95% submitted within 90 days	Internal standard	100%	100%	100%	95%	100%

Figure 8.2 Example of a transplant dashboard–kidney transplant.

Do: Carry out the changes on a small scale, document the problems, and gather data.

Study: Analyze data and summarize learnings.

Act: Repeat cycle if results were unsuccessful, modify plan if results were partially successful, or hardwire practices if entirely successful [4].

Figure 8.3 is a diagrammatic rendering of the cycle which repeats over and over until the desired results are achieved. Figure 8.4 shows several examples of transplant-specific PDSA performance improvement initiatives.

Once the performance improvement team has completed the analysis of the area of improvement and generated a solution, this solution must be placed into practice and must have a mechanism to ensure that the solution is sustained. Usually, this is accomplished through periodic audits of records or charts or through the comparison with benchmarks until there is confidence that new practices are hardwired into the program or organization.

Sentinel and adverse events

Unfortunately, unforeseen and unintentional adverse events do occur during the management of all patients, including transplant patients. Adverse events are those patient management errors that result in harm to the patient. There are also "near misses" where an error is made; however, it is caught in time and no harm is caused to the patient. Significant adverse events are called "sentinel events" and defined as an "unexpected

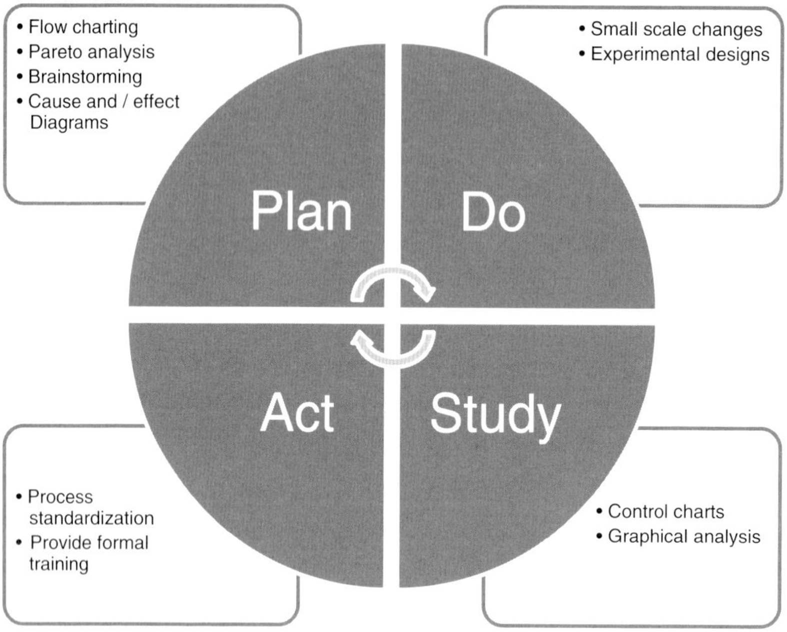

Figure 8.3 PDSA cycle.

occurrence involving death or serious physical or psychological injury, or the risk thereof" [5].

Adverse events are usually caused by many interrelated factors, some systemic or related to the organization and/or process and some due to human error. In studying adverse events, most were caused by systemic failures, specifically, poor communications, lack of safeguards, and lack of

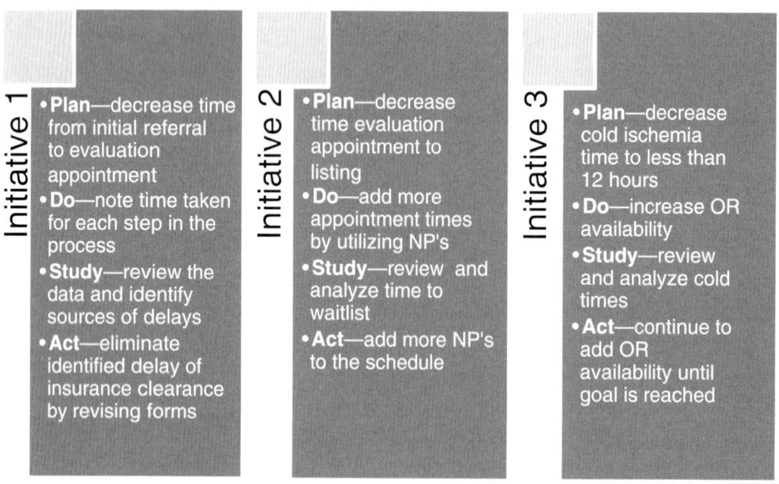

Figure 8.4 PDSA examples.

resources. Human error also plays a role where lack of training and knowledge, failure to follow procedures, fatigue, and overwork, all contribute to adverse outcomes. Examples of adverse events in transplantation are

- transplant of organs into unintended recipients;
- living donor organs retrieved but not transplanted;
- living donor death and organ failure;
- living donor who within 2 years of donation is listed for a liver or a kidney;
- ABO incompatibility of donor and recipient (unless intended);
- unintended transmission of infectious agents to a recipient.

When an adverse event is identified, the transplant center must document the event and notify the OPTN. In the case of transmission of infectious agents from a donor to recipients, it must be reported to the OPO and the OPTN Patient Safety System [6]. The response and the timeliness of response to this event is critical since the risks of not doing so are many: potential hazard to other recipients, sends a mixed message regarding the importance of patient safety to staff, increases likelihood of lawsuits and regulatory actions, invites media scrutiny, and decreases overall patient trust [7]. The center must conduct an analysis of why the event occurred and will use this analysis to effect changes in policies and practices to prevent repeat incidents. CMS regulations state:

> "A transplant center must establish and implement written policies to address and document adverse events that occur during any phase of an organ transplantation case. The policies must address at a minimum, the process for the identification, reporting, analysis and prevention of adverse events." (CFR 482.96)

The most common methodology to investigate an adverse event is a root-cause analysis (RCA), which is a process used to discern the underlying reasons for an adverse event in order to prevent the recurrence of a harmful outcome or a near miss. The Joint Commission now requires a RCA be performed for all sentinel events. There is no one way to perform a RCA; however, it usually begins with the following steps:

1. Collection of data concerning the event.
2. Assembling a team to conduct the investigation. These individuals could be from the transplant program, quality department, or a combination of both.
3. Flow charting of the chain of events, identifying where in the chain of events that the process broke down and the causal factors.
4. Developing a cause-and-effect diagram in order to drill down to the root causes.
5. Generating recommendations for improvement and development of risk-reduction strategies.

A number of tools can be employed to assist with the analysis such as cause and effect charting, fishbone diagramming, or use of the five whys. References for a more in-depth discussion on the use of these tools can be found in the bibliography. The Joint Commission has reviewed several thousand sentinel events that have occurred in their accredited organizations and have found the top three root causes are poor communication, poor assessment of a patient's physical or emotional condition, and lack of orientation or training [8]. The UNOS Operations and Safety Committee identified that 38% of all transplant adverse events were caused by mislabeling and packaging [9]. Once the root cause or causes have been identified, there must be specific actions taken to prevent a repeat occurrence. These have been termed risk-reduction strategies by The Joint Commission and can be broadly grouped into three categories:

- Reduce the chance of failure.
- Help staff correctly perform their duties.
- Assist staff in recognizing errors before harm is done [10].

A simple checklist is a tool that can provide powerful results in decreasing errors. Dr. Peter Pronovost, from Johns Hopkins University, decreased ICU infections by 70% by developing a checklist for providers [11]. Checklists are also useful in transplant programs both for quality and for regulatory reasons, as seen in Figure 8.5. The last step in the RCA process is to ensure that the strategy is implemented, tested, and formalized. This is typically accomplished through a change in policy or procedures with the subsequent communication and training to staff.

Recently, cumulative sum or CUSUM has been utilized by the SRTR to provide transplant centers with a more proactive approach to monitoring post-transplant outcomes. CUSUM methodologies allow real-time monitoring of a process so that changes are quickly identified and, if problematic, can be resolved. The method was first developed in the 1950s and has been increasingly used in recent years in the healthcare arena.

The CUSUM method, basically explained, begins with values or measurements being obtained on a process. The difference between each data point and an identified benchmark is then calculated and summed up. If the process is "in control," collected data will not show much deviation around the benchmark value and in theory, the data above the benchmark value and the data below the benchmark value will average each other out. However, if the process is out of control, the data will be to one side of the benchmark and the CUSUM chart will clearly show that deviation. It is particularly useful in identifying small changes and trends in processes. The SRTR has begun to provide each transplant center with CUSUM charts for their own transplant program which shows post-transplant survival outcomes in real time. This tool should be understood and used

Patient education checklist for kidney transplant

- ☐ Patient explained the irreversibility of CKD and that transplant is not a cure
- ☐ Reviewed the etiology of CKD and the effect on transplant
- ☐ Reviewed deceased donor transplant including wait time, risks, expanded donor criteria, DCD
- ☐ Reviewed living donor transplant including related vs. non related, benefits, donor suitability criteria, evaluation process for donors
- ☐ Reviewed transplant program's current graft and patient survival statistics
- ☐ Explained HLA typing and panel reactive antibody
- ☐ Explained evaluation testing and the reasons for performing tests
- ☐ Explained the surgical procedure
- ☐ Explained delayed graft function including symptoms and treatment
- ☐ Explained the most common infectious agents
- ☐ Explained the potential impact of organ donor risk factors on a successful outcome
- ☐ Explained that graft failure will result in the return to dialysis
- ☐ Explained immunosuppressive agents, the reason for taking, the side effects both short and long term
- ☐ Explained what to expect during the transplant hospitalization
- ☐ Explained the usual schedule for post transplant clinic visits and laboratories /
- ☐ Explained how much time to take off from work
- ☐ Explained the importance of financial preparedness and the risks
- ☐ All questions answered

Figure 8.5 Example of checklist.

by each program in order to develop a more robust and timely QAPI program.

A more proactive approach to quality and patient safety is to utilize failure mode and effects analysis (FMEA). This method is used to identify when, where, and how processes might fail. It emphasizes prevention rather than reacting to problems or adverse conditions. FMEA is made up of four steps:

- Failure modes (what could go wrong?)
- Failure causes (why would the failure happen?)
- Failure effects (what would be the consequences of each failure?)
- Failure prevention (how can we prevent a bad result when there is a failure?)

Identifying areas within the transplant program where there is risk for adverse events or gaps in care which may lead to poor patient outcomes is where this method is particularly helpful. It has been estimated that there are 48 handoffs from organ procurement to beginning the transplant surgery [12]. Given the sheer number of handoffs, the process is predisposed for an error to occur. An example of a simplified tool to assist in developing the FMEA is the worksheet shown in Table 8.3 [13].

Table 8.3 FMEA worksheet example

Function	Potential failure mode	Potential effect of failure	Potential cause of failure	Current process controls	Recommended action	Responsibility	Action taken
Patient not waitlisted in a timely manner	Patient did not get scheduled	Dissatisf ed referring physicians and patients	Poor communication. Lack of staff backup when out of office	None	Use of check off list to ensure all patients are scheduled	Clinical manager	
	Testing not completed	Delay in waitlisting	Deficit in patient education and follow-up	None	Follow-up with patient every month. Stress importance of testing in patient education sessions	Coordinators	
	Testing inconclusive, retesting needed	Increased cost to patient	Laboratory test sensitivity, sampling error	None	Evaluate other laboratory test methodologies if available	Laboratory manager	

Last, the hallmark of an organization that is dedicated to clinical excellence is nurturance of a culture of quality and performance improvement. This culture is fostered first at the top of the organization through senior leaders, who stress the importance of quality to employees and physicians, to maintain an atmosphere of empowerment and transparency, and to provide the resources necessary to sustain a quality culture. The transplant program thus becomes a beneficiary of this quality culture where the program is supported within the larger confines of the organization. Failure to attain this quality culture will have dire consequences to the organization and the transplant program. Program viability could hang in the balance. Regulatory consequences are discussed in Chapter 5.

References

1 U.S. Department of Health and Human Services. Health Resources and Services Administration. 2007. The HRSA Transplant Center Growth and Management Collaborative Best Practices Final Report. p. x.
2 Catapult Consultants, LLC. Quality Assessment and Performance Improvement (QAPI) Programs: A Resource Guide for Transplant Surveyors. 2010.
3 University Health System Consortium. 2004. Transplant Services. 2003 Benchmarking Project Field Book.
4 Spath P. *Introduction to Healthcare Quality Management.* Chicago: Health Administration.
5 Joint Commission on Accreditation of Healthcare Organizations. Sentinel events: evaluating cause and planning improvement. 1998. Library of congress catalog number 97-80531.
6 OPTN Policy 4.3: Disclosure of Post-Transplant Discovery Of Donor Disease or Malignancy and Notification of Recipients.
7 Conway J, Federico F, Stewart K, Campbell M. *Respectful Management of Serious Clinical Adverse Events (Second Edition).* IHI Innovation Series white paper. Cambridge, Massachusetts: Institute for Healthcare Improvement; 2011.
8 The Joint Commission. 2007. Improving America's Hospitals: The Joint Commission's Annual Report on Quality and Safety, 2007.
9 Pondrom S. Check and Recheck. The AJT Report. *Am J Transplant.* 2011;11:1346.
10 Spath P. *Introduction to Healthcare Quality Management.* Chicago: Health Administration Press; 2009: p. 195.
11 Pronovost P. *Safe Patients, Smart Hospitals: How One Doctor's Checklist Can Help Us Change Health Care from the Inside Out.* New York: Hudson Street Press; 2010.
12 Steinberger D, Douglas SV, Kirschbaum MS. Use of failure mode and effects analysis for proactive identification of communication and handoff failures from organ procurement to transplantation. *Prog Transplant.* 19;3:208–214.
13 Tauge N. *The Quality Toolbox.* Milwaukee: ASQ Quality Press; 2004. pp. 236–240.

CHAPTER 9

Transplant Information Management and Transplant Information Systems

Lauren E. Kearns
Transplant Services, University of North Carolina Medical Center, Center for Transplant Care, Chapel Hill, NC, USA

Solid organ transplantation is a highly data-intensive field of healthcare. Transplant centers use health-related data collected about patients for their direct and individualized care and for outcomes analysis and management, quality assessment and performance improvement, business process analysis, contracting, research, and a host of other clinical and non-clinical activities. The information needs of the twenty-first-century transplant center are now so extensive and highly regulated that transplant centers must adopt advanced computer-assisted methodologies to manage their data and information. With each passing day, it becomes less likely that a transplant center, even a small one, can manage their data and information needs using paper-based systems. In this chapter, we will gain an understanding of data, information, and knowledge look at the history behind data management in transplantation, the tools and methodologies available to transplant centers, advances in the rapidly changing electronic health record (EHR) landscape, and the driving forces for data management in the transplant center today.

Data, information, knowledge, and wisdom (DIKW)

It is a good idea to step back now to provide some background and definitions that are meaningful to the transplant environment for data and information management. This will help the reader to more fully appreciate and understand the environment from the macroscopic and microscopic viewpoints.

Data, information, knowledge, and wisdom (DIKW) are often seen as a continuum of increasing complexity and inter-relationships. This DIKW

Transplant Administration, First Edition. Edited by Lisa Norris.

Companion website: www.wiley.com/go/norris/transplantadmin

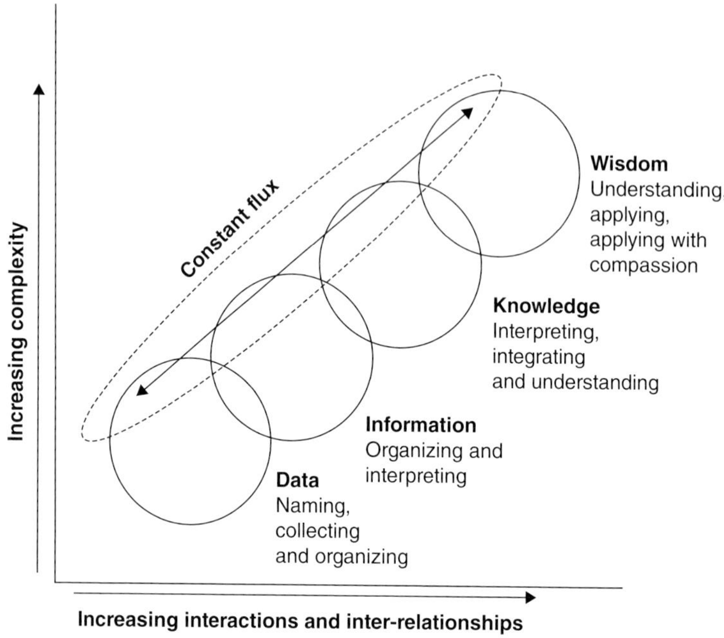

Figure 9.1 The relationship of data, information, knowledge, and wisdom.
Source: This figure is a modification from a figure originally printed in Englebardt S. and Nelson R. (2002). *Health Care Informatics: An Interdisciplinary Approach*. This version of the figure is designed by Ramona Nelson and printed here with the permission of Ramona Nelson.

model by Nelson [1] demonstrates the inter-relatedness of the four concepts as seen in Figure 9.1.

History of regulated transplant data collection

Transplant data collection as a regulatory requirement began in the United States with the interpretation of the National Organ Transplant Act (NOTA) of 1984 as discussed in Chapter 1. The Scientific Registry for Transplant Recipients (SRTR) was established in 1987 as a national computerized database to analyze all data collected by the Organ Procurement Transplantation Network (OPTN) and report on the effectiveness of transplantation in the United States. The SRTR provided the first national clinical research database for organ transplantation [2]. A timeline of milestones in data reporting is depicted in Figure 9.2. From 1987 to 2007, the SRTR's capabilities for collecting, analyzing, and reporting data grew significantly with the advancement of computing technology. In turn, the responsibility of the transplant center to understand and respond to reported outcomes also increased, which amplified the need to have better

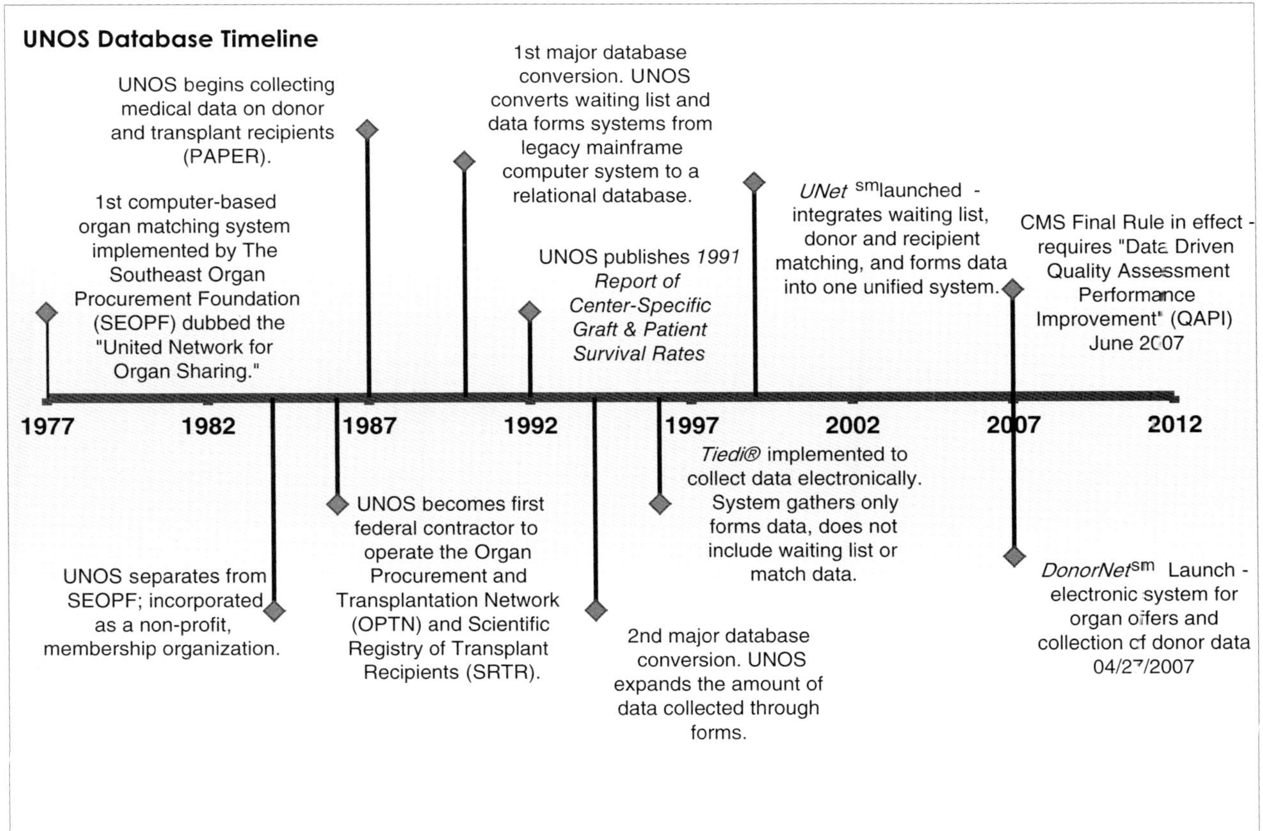

Figure 9.2 Data timeline.
Source: Data from the United Network for Organ Sharing. *History of Database*. http://www.unos.org/donation/ index.php?topic=history of database *(accessed September 10, 2012)*. [2,3]

tools for data collection and analysis and performance improvement. In 2007, the transplant world underwent a transformation primarily due to the new CMS requirements to meet clinical outcomes performance standards and establish robust QAPI programs [4].

The lagging state of computerization in health care

The success in developing a scientific registry was highly dependent on advances in computer technology; the scientific community and the business community were early adopters to this technology, while health care for clinical purposes was not. During the late 1980s and early 1990s, while many health care entities had installed computerized billing and registration systems, very few had clinical systems. The computerized patient record (CPR), the predecessor of today's electronic health record (EHR), made its appearance in some US hospitals at the end of the 1960s and early 1970s, but its use and adoption remained quite limited for several decades [5]. In actuality, most of these first-generation hospital clinical systems were typically little more than computerized order entry communication systems where a clinician or a clerk would select a patient name from a census and then order a test, a diet, or a piece of equipment, and the order was sent to the receiving department. Order entry systems were replaced by order processing systems that incorporated two-way communication and status updates; once the ordering department had completed the test, a communication was sent back to indicate the status of the test, for example, COM (complete). In time, clinical system functionality included results; a verified order would send back an electronic message about results—"Creatinine 2.4 mg/dL—High." The major purpose of these clinical order systems was to communicate orders from one department to another and capture charges for patient billing [5].

Another drawback to early clinical systems was that they were frequently "stand-alone" systems, meaning that other than sharing a common registration system for census, they were not connected to other hospital systems (interfaced) and therefore these systems did not "talk" to each other. When a notification came back on the order entry system to indicate that the laboratory test results were available, the user would need to look in the laboratory computer system to see the results. Users may not have had direct access to the laboratory system to look up results; instead they relied on printed or faxed results from the hospital laboratory. Different types of data were housed in separate information silos.

Early clinical systems also had the disadvantage of being very difficult for the average user to access in terms of pulling data out of the system (data mining). Mainframe computers systems were very large, expensive, and required professionally trained computer personnel to operate them

[5]. Most clinical users had neither physical access nor the programming skills required to create a query to extract data. Requests for data required formal work orders and sometimes weeks of waiting for reports from the hospital information technology (IT) group. Many of these systems also did not have mechanisms for long-term storage [5]. Early hospital systems typically were of limited use when it came to the increasing regulatory demands for collecting, analyzing, and acting on a center's transplant data.

The need for data management in the transplant center

A transplant center needs an efficient and effective method to collect and store data so that information is useable immediately, available to all personnel for direct clinical care, and retrievable at any future time for secondary use. Having the right tools and processes for data collection and storage is foundational to the success of the transplant center. Without a sophisticated electronic clinical record, most transplant centers have had to establish processes that either were outside the hospital system or are run in parallel to meet workflow and regulatory reporting needs.

The referral and evaluation

The collection of transplant data begins with the patient referral for transplant evaluation. This document is a rich source of data and information for the transplant center. Establishing a standardized and consistent methodology for referral intake (and for all data management processes) will help to ensure reliable and valid program data.

A complete transplant referral should contain all the necessary patient data to begin multiple processes at once. The clinical process requires a preliminary assessment of a patient's potential eligibility to meet the center's standard transplant candidacy criteria, for example, age, height and weight, diagnosis related to end-stage organ failure and date of onset, all comorbidities, a current medication list, surgical history, any history of substance abuse, or malignancy, in addition to recent results of all laboratory and procedural/radiological testing.

The referral also should contain all the data elements needed for business processes to begin: date of referral, name, date of birth, social security number (SSN) (still required by UNOS), home address, including county and zip code, local address if temporarily re-locating for transplant, contact numbers of patient and family (work, home, cell), the referring physician's name and contact info, the patient's insurance carrier, policy number, group number, guarantor, and if the referral is made by the insurance case manager the authorization and dates approved for the transplant evaluation.

Without integrated information systems, a transplant center would need to create manual processes for referral intake and data management. Transplant Nurse Coordinators might be responsible for developing organ specific forms to capture referral information and to summarize the results of the comprehensive multidisciplinary evaluation. As the patient moved through the evaluation process, data were collected and recorded manually on these forms, which were then stored in the transplant office "shadow chart." It is highly likely that this compilation of patient information, which may have come from the patient's primary care provider or a specialist (e.g., a vaccination record, a colonoscopy report, or a dental clearance form), never became part of the patient's official medical record, instead it was stored in the shadow chart in the transplant office; making the shadow chart a very valuable, but physically isolated or "silo-ed" resource.

Post-transplant

The post-transplant phase of care is typically structured around clinical encounters, such as labs, visits, and hospitalizations. The ledger sized paper flow chart with multiple rows and columns, would be initiated when the newly transplanted patient was in the ICU. It literally followed the patient for their post-transplant lifetime; wherever the patient was located, inpatient or outpatient, the flowchart followed. These documents held near sacred status—they contained every laboratory test result, from both external laboratories and transplant center laboratories, every immunosuppression (IS) dose change, every biopsy result, and every intervention initiated for the post-transplant patient. The flow chart is representative of the difference in care for transplant patients. Most patient care is episodic; transplant care is provided across a continuum. Like the referral intake form, the flow chart, rarely became part of the patient's official record, yet it contained the most complete picture of the transplant patient in one document.

The data required to complete UNOS forms, for example, the Transplant Candidate Registration (TCR) or Transplant Recipient Form (TRF), were often hand-compiled from these shadow charts and flowcharts by clerical personnel (data coordinators) and/or nurses. In the past all forms were mailed, then faxed to UNOS. Now, web-based electronic data entry through Transplant Information Electronic Data Interchange (TIEDI®) is the standard. Only a few clinical transplant information systems have the functionality to transmit data directly from the transplant system to UNOS, thereby eliminating manual data entry.

Due to the lagging nature that persists in the adoption of EHRs and the lack of a fully integrated record that completely meets the business and clinical needs of the transplant center, many transplant practices continue to operate using paper records or hybrid systems, for example, both electronic and paper, for some processes.

The problem with paper

Practices such as these highlight the intrinsic problems with paper-based patient records for both patient care and data management. Paper records create physical and intellectual silos, which may have a negative effect on patient care and business practices in multiple ways:

- *Inaccessibility*—paper records require that the user come to where the record is located. Only one person can access the record at one time, and records are not available at the user's convenience (24/7). Complex and inconvenient processes are required to access paper records—for example, records must be checked out from the Medical Records Department [5]. Physical inaccessibility or "silo-ing" of medical data perpetuates the need for transplant staff to create "shadow charts" or copies of the original record that are housed where the staff are and where the data is easily accessible. The convenience of shadow charts creates other issues, such as unintentional housing of original documentation creating problems with medical record integrity.
- *Lack of Integration in Clinical Care*—paper records that are physically inaccessible also create intellectual silos. Paper records limit the integration of the multidisciplinary team approach to care. For example, a paper-based consultation may require the addition of several steps for information transfer to occur, for example, a telephone call from one provider to another to share information already recorded on paper. Moreover, the results of the discussion between these providers, perhaps a new diagnosis or treatment plan change, may not be captured at all, and is therefore information that is unavailable to other caregivers, current and future. Paper records may prevent transplant clinicians from knowing on a timely basis that the patient was seen by nontransplant health care providers. For example, yesterday a patient was seen in the transplant clinic and had a medication change. The patient develops a fever overnight, but their record is in medical records and unavailable when they present to the emergency department (ED). The ED physician is not aware of the medication change, nor will the transplant provider be made aware that the ED physician has prescribed an antibiotic that requires IS dose reduction. It may be days or several weeks before this information is discovered serendipitously, when the patient's monthly labs show decreased renal function and supratherapeutic IS trough levels.
- *Issues with Data Integrity and Accuracy*—paper records require that transplant administrative support personnel spend a large percentage of their

work time transcribing source document data, for example, manually recording patient laboratory reports onto a paper flowchart. This process is prone to transcription errors such as numerical transposition, and errors due to "data fatigue" may occur, such as "wrong record–wrong data." Incorrect data or illegible handwriting may cause harm to the patient at the time, and, if left uncorrected, can create future harm as well. If incorrect data are used for research or clinical outcomes management, then this data is not representative of the care that the patient has received, nor does it accurately represent their response to treatment.

- *Limited Capabilities for Statistical Analysis and Quality Improvement*—paper records require manual extraction and auditing for quality reporting and statistical analysis. Data found in paper records are not automatically reusable, which decreases efficiency. Paper-based processes for statistical analysis and Quality Assessment and Performance Improvement (QAPI) are labor intensive, and difficult to replicate, manipulate, or analyze for both individual and population-based outcomes and reporting.

The scope of transplant care and regulatory reporting is for the lifetime of the patient and/or the graft; this requires a data management system that is able to capture essential pre- and post-transplant data, store it longitudinally, and make it easily retrievable and reusable.

Spreadsheet and database applications

The creation of smaller, or personal, computers (PCs) based on silicon chip technology revolutionized computer technology [6]. Smaller computers cost less and did not require professionally trained programmers to operate them. In the 1980s, programs like IBM's *Lotus 1-2-3* and *Excel* from Microsoft Office became commercially available. These "spreadsheet" applications presented data in a table-type format for organization and analysis and included arithmetical and statistical functionality, as well as graphing and charting capability. Designed to look like the familiar accounting ledger of multiple columns and rows, these tools were readily adopted in transplant centers and continue to be used heavily today, to capture manually entered data and store it for future analysis. Data, stored in these "flat files" or single spreadsheet tables, were readily available, easily retrievable, and reusable. As an example, one spreadsheet file might include all the data elements related to all the transplants performed in one year (see Table 9.1).

Spreadsheet applications act like simple databases in terms of storage, organization, and retrieval, but they lack true database functionality and sophistication. "A formal *database* is a structured collection of individual data elements... A *database management system (DBMS)* is a software program that is used to manage, organize, and retrieve data and

Table 9.1 An example of a simple spreadsheet for all transplants performed in 2012

Name_Last	Name_First	MRN	Tx_Date	Tx_Type	Tx_Surgeon	Procuring_ Surgeon
St. John	Deborah	1234567-8	4/15/2012	Heart	Chapel	North
Spartan	Lori	2468024-6	10/10/2012	Kidney	Hill	Jordan
Ricardo	Alessandra	1357913-5	6/1/2012	Lung	North	Chapel
Joseph	Michael	131313-9	1/19/2012	Liver	Jordan	Hill

information from a database" [7]. A DBMS is much more powerful than a spreadsheet application, because it is designed to permit complex query functionality across many related tables within the database. The *relational database* contains data stored in multiple tables that may be related or linked. That is, each "type" of data element has its own table, compared to the spreadsheet application which stores all the data in one file. To yield the same information about annual transplants (Table 9.1) requires a "query" that will pull specific information from three different tables in a relational database (Table 9.2). Commercial DBMS programs, for example, Microsoft Office Access, Oracle, and SQL (Structured Query Language), became an indispensable component in the transplant toolset to manage data and information.

Data that are organized in a table format are easy to locate, sort, and perform computations on. For instance, using the data in the Patient table, we can create fields in the table to calculate the age at transplant for each patient as well as the number of days that each patient is "post-transplant." Manipulating or querying the tables in the database can produce unlimited reports for clinical and business functions. Despite the lack of sophisticated mainframe clinical systems to capture, store, and easily retrieve data, with personal computers and their software applications, transplant centers developed their own databases to manage the myriad of regulatory reporting needs, analyze clinical patient outcomes, and perform business functions and still rely heavily on these methods of data management.

In lieu of a computerized record system, a database system could be created as a repository for all transplant data, for example, referrals, and pre- and post-transplant clinical data. Databases provided transplant centers with a greater degree of control over their business and clinical data and, unlike mainframe computers, did not require the skills of a professional programmer. At least one "computer-savvy" person who knew or could learn how to use the database was needed to build tables and forms and write queries to extract data. Data entry could be done by clerical or clinical personnel. Transplant centers were able to independently produce information necessary for clinical outcomes management and regulatory reporting.

Table 9.2 The patient, surgeon, and organ type tables

Patient Table

MRN	Name_Last	Name_First	DOB	Address	City	State	Tx_Date
X23457-8	St. John	Deborah	1/1/1957	33604 Oak St.	Flushing	NY	4/15/2012
X46804-6	Spartan	Lori	4/15/1977	1 Chocolate Lane	Hershey	PA	10/1/2012
X35793-5	Ricardo	Alessandra	5/10/1985	455 Green St.	Lizard Lick	NC	6/1/2012
X31313-9	Joseph	Michael	10/7/1975	461 Ocean Blvd.	Jupiter	FL	1/19/2012

Surgeon Table

ID_Number	Surgeon_Name	UPIN
C123	Chapel	C123456
H456	Hill	H456789
N789	North	N987654
J258	Jordan	J321654

Organ Type Table

ID_Number	Organ_Type
1	Heart
2	Lung
3	Liver
4	Kidney
5	Pancreas
6	Intestine

In 1988, the University of Pittsburgh was one of the first transplant centers to publically report on the development of a center-designed computerized database for kidney transplant—Transplant Information Management System (TIMY) [8]. The TIMY database was built on an IBM computer with a 30-megabyte hard-drive. Just think, today, that is less than one-twentieth of what a compact disc (CD) can hold, and one recordable DVD disc is 150 times bigger than the IBM computer hard-drive that held the TIMY database.

TIMY was designed to store manually entered information about all phases of transplant (pre-, peri-, and post-op follow-up care). To make the database more user friendly, a number of data fields had built in precoded choices for faster data entry. Reports were preconfigured, for example, the weekly listing of candidates, and other reports could be designed as needed. Every patient was entered into the database, creating an individual patient record. A waiting list composite scoring system was designed to facilitate organ offer matching between candidates and donors. Data used for this report included total waiting time, HLA match, the panel-reactive antibody (PRA) status, the patient's medical urgency, and their logistics information such as how far the patient was from the center or if they were in-house. Nurses used laptops loaded with TIMY to manage organ offers after normal work hours. In addition to clinical care, the database was used for research, and business reporting needs, such as insurance company information requests [8]. In 1988, this was a very innovative system. Figure 9.3 depicts a TIMY form used to capture candidate information.

For many years, these "home grown" database solutions served the transplant center's needs well, but because they relied on manual data entry, and did not have the capability to automatically capture data from the hospital's computerized registration system or laboratory system, their value remained limited. The full potential of a database could be more fully realized when it could be combined with the ability to automatically receive and capture data from the data source, eliminating inefficient, error-prone, and time-consuming manual intervention.

Developing transplant-specific electronic records

Throughout the 1990s and early 2000s, EHR implementation in the United States played out much more slowly than expected. This was attributed to a number of issues: the high cost of purchase, implementation and maintenance of EHR applications, poor financial incentives for providers, highly publicized history of costly but failed efforts, and growing concerns about confidentiality and security [9]. As transplant centers grew in both the numbers of patients requiring transplantation, and the volume of

TRANSPLANT INFORMATION MANAGEMENT SYSTEM - KIDNEY REGISTRY - DEMOGRAPHICS

****

ID# ____________ LAST NAME ____________ FIRST NAME ____________

DATE OF BIRTH ____________

SEX ________ RACE ____________

BLOOD GROUP ABO ________ RH ________ LEWIS ANTIGEN A _____ B ___

HLA TYPE A ___ . ___B___ . ___Bw___DR___ . ___DQ___ . ___DRw___ . ___ TISSUS TYPING # ____

DIAGNOSIS ____________

DATE DIAGNOSIS WAS FIRST MADE ____________

COMMENT ____________

****

IF PATIENT LOST TO FOLLOW-UP, ENTER DATE OF LAST FOLLOW-UP ____________

IF PATIENT DIED, ENTER DATE OF DEATH ____________

PRIMARY CAUSE OF DEATH ____________

SECONDARY CAUSES OF DEATH

2. ____________
3. ____________
4. ____________
5. ____________

COMMENT ____________

****

Fig2. Every pationt ontered in the TIMY kidney transplant management system has a lartinent record demopraphic date. Most of the date is entered in precoded choice fields, which minimizes date entry arrors and greatly facilitates later analysis

TRANSPLANT INFORMATION MANAGEMENT SYSTEM-KIDNEY REGISTRY-CANDIDATE DATE

****

ID# ____________ LAST NAME ____________ FIRST ____________

CURRENT RECORD ___ CANDIDACY FOR GRAFT # ___ ABO ______ ALIEN _____

PHYSICIAN CODE ______ DIALYSIS CENTER CODE ______ SEND LETTER _____

DATE REFERRED ________ PREFERENCE ____________

LIST STATUS ____________ URGENCY ________ LOGISTICS ______

INSURANCE ____________ SECONDARY ____________

AGE ______ AGE GROUP ________ TOTAL PREGNANCIES ______ LIVE BIRTHS ___

HEIGHT ___ ft ___ in OR ___ cm

PRA HIGHEST _____ DATE _____ PRA RECENT _____ DATE _____

HAAb _____ HBsAg _____ HBsAb ______ HBcAb ______

CMV ______ HIV ELISA TESTING _____ WESTERN BLOT ___

PRE-KTX BLOOD TRANSFUSIONS WHOLE BLOOD ______ PACKED RED CELLS _____

WASHED CELLS ___ FROZEN/FILTERED PLASMA _____ PLATELETS ___ BUFFY COATS ___

IF LIVING DONOR. ENTER # OF DONOR SPECIFIC TRANSFUSIONS ________

DATE OF LAST PRE-KTY TRANSFUSION ____________

START OF DIALYSIS ____________ TYPE ____________

NEPHRECTOMY ____________ DATE ________ REASON ________

SPLENECTOMY ____________ DATE ________

ADDITIONAL DIAGNOSIS

HEPATIC ____________
PULMONARY ____________
CARDIOVASCULAR ____________
JUVENILE DIABETES MELLITUS ____________
ADULT DIABETES MELLITUS ____________
DITABETIC TREATMENT ____________

COMMENTS ____________

****

Figure 9.3 Candidate form in TIMY.

Source: Markus BH, Mitchell S, Gordon RD, Gillauist B, Tzakis AG, Starzl TE. TIMY-A Center-Oriented Transplant Information. *Transplantation Proceedings*. 1998;20(1)1, Suppl. 1:385–390. Reproduced with permission of Elsevier.

transplants performed, manual processes became increasingly inefficient, and ineffective [8].

Those transplant centers whose parent organizations (e.g., the hospital) did implement large enterprise wide systems found that no matter how robust the system for general needs, it was often a poor fit for the transplant center because of differences in workflows, as well as clinical, regulatory, and business data needs. These "super-sized–one size fits all" systems were designed to fit the majority of care that a patient received, which by and large was episodic in nature, and thus a generic approach was required. Unfortunately, the "super-sized" approach lacks the customization that specialized chronic disease medical programs like organ transplantation require. Transplant care is longitudinal with multiple subspecialties working in concert to provide an individualized approach for each organ system.

While many centers continued to use paper-based documentation, supplemented by manual data capture spreadsheet applications, several innovative transplant centers successfully developed more sophisticated interfaced databases and turned them into successful commercial products. These niche applications were like mini-EHRs—they had a graphical user interface (GUI) that included icons, menus, and dialog boxes on the screen, and they were interoperable, having the ability to bidirectionally exchange simple data across an interface without losing data integrity. By connecting to existing computerized systems via an electronic interface, they automatically received and stored data such as patient demographics, laboratory results, text-based data and reports, and admission transfer and discharge (ADT) data, and in turn they could electronically transmit data to the parent EHR as well as upload formatted and batched data about multiple patients to UNOS for regulatory reporting, eliminating the need for separate manual processes for regulatory reporting.

These transplant information systems had built-in functionality tailored to the transplant workflow, and the multidisciplinary team could see and care for the patient using a "transplant lens." For example, external labs were documented alongside the internal hospital labs, just like in the paper flowchart, providing a complete picture of the patient's IS levels and renal function. Patient referrals and patient progress through the evaluation was tracked electronically and transplant centers could quickly measure their median "Referral to Waitlist" times. Waitlist functionality as well as organ-specific tools, such as the MELD-PELD calculator, were embedded in the software, providing instantaneous and effortless access to reports, e.g., total transplants performed for the current year or for the past 10 years became an effortless task that required minimal training. The database itself became a valued and irreplaceable resource. Any piece of data that had been assigned a field in the database, for example, transplant date, organ type, transplanting surgeon, donor age, donor cause of death, cold ischemic time, transplant type, laterality, CMV status, etc., was easily retrievable, and made outcome analysis and research, easier to manage

ROI	Initial costs	Year 2	Year 3	Year 4	Year 5	Total
System purchase (included data migration)	$350K	NA	NA	NA	NA	$350K
Annual maintenance	NA	$30K	$30K	$30K	$30K	$120K
Salaries	$100K	$100K	$100K	$100K	$100K	$500K
Total expenses	$450K	$130K	$130K	$130K	$130K	$970K
Total of year 1 and year 2	$580K					
Salaries required if no system purchased	$300K	$300K	$300K	$300K	$300K	$1.5 Million
Total of year 1 and year 2	$600K					(5 Year savings = $530K)

Figure 9.4 Return on investment for the purchase of a transplant database in 2003.

and much more accurate. Arguably, these niche applications transformed the work of the transplant center and its staff.

While these smaller niche systems were less expensive than enterprise-wide EHRs, they were not cheap. One transplant center leveraged the purchase of their transplant system by comparing the purchase and start-up costs of the transplant system to the person-hours required to do manual data collection and regulatory reporting for the next 5 years. This model of return-on-investment demonstrated that the system would pay for itself in 2 years, and the resources gained, such as compliance with timely regulatory reporting, plus the database itself as a repository were priceless [personal experience]. See Figure 9.4.

The current EHR environment

In February 2009, the Health Information Technology for Economic and Clinical Health (HITECH) Act was signed into law as a part of the 2009 American Recovery and Reinvestment Act (ARRA). The goal of HITECH was to promote "the adoption and meaningful use of health information technology" [10]. The HITECH Act defines an EHR as "an electronic record of health-related information on an individual that is created, gathered, managed, and consulted by authorized health care clinicians and staff" (Section 13400(5)) [11]. Powerful financial incentives are available for those institutions that choose to adopt early, and significant financial disincentives (i.e., decreased Medicare payments) will be administered to those who do not. This financially driven regulatory landscape has created a feverish drive for certified EHR purchase and implementation across the nation which may create new problems for the transplant administrator.

One concern about the system-wide EHR is that it "may not be of the proper granulation of data, whereas a (niche system) represents a specialized view of the data optimized to the ... (specialist's) needs" [12]. A recent survey of the transplant administrator's list serv group (TransplantAdministrators@yahoogroups.com) reveals that despite EHR fever, most certified EHR systems do not adequately address the specific needs of transplantation, requiring transplant centers to continue to use niche-type systems for "registry" needs (clinical and outcomes research, and regulatory reporting) if they have them, while others continue to rely on paper-based methods and non-integrated spreadsheets. Perhaps, the future state of a fully integrated electronic health information exchange (HIE) that connects all EHRs across the nation will negate the duplicate and hybrid processes we have had to develop to manage data collection, analysis, and reporting. When that time comes, CMS and the OPTN may be able to pull their required data at regular intervals, eliminating a very large data burden on transplant centers, but until then transplant professionals will continue to use whatever systems are available to collect and manage data, provide evidenced-based care, and to create knowledge about their patient populations.

Living and dying by the SRTR

In 1987, NOTA set forth the law that mandated the development of the SRTR; so much has happened in the quarter century since then. Today, the SRTR provides national comprehensive and comparative reporting and analytics of all aggregated transplant data by center, by region, and nationally. This data is used for many purposes including research and regulatory enforcement [4]. The SRTR database contains nearly 30 years worth of rich data about the full range of transplant activity—transplant candidates, organ donors, transplant recipients, and their survival. The SRTR participates in transplant policy development by providing thorough data analysis to make evidence-based decisions [4]. In addition to data collected directly from transplant centers by the OPTN (e.g., via the myriad of forms, such as the TCR, Transplant Recipient Registration (TRR), or TRF), a number of other data sources are used by the SRTR, i.e., Social Security Death Master File (SSDMF), the CMS–End-Stage Renal Disease (ESRD) database, CMS claims data, the National Death Index (NDI), Surveillance Epidemiology and End Results (SEER), the American Hospital Association (AHA), and the National Center for Health Statistics (NCHS) [13]. The data flow and the data sources are depicted in Figure 9.5.

SRTR program-specific reports

The SRTR prepares and publishes program-specific reports (PSRs) for every organ transplant program in the United States twice a year, in January and

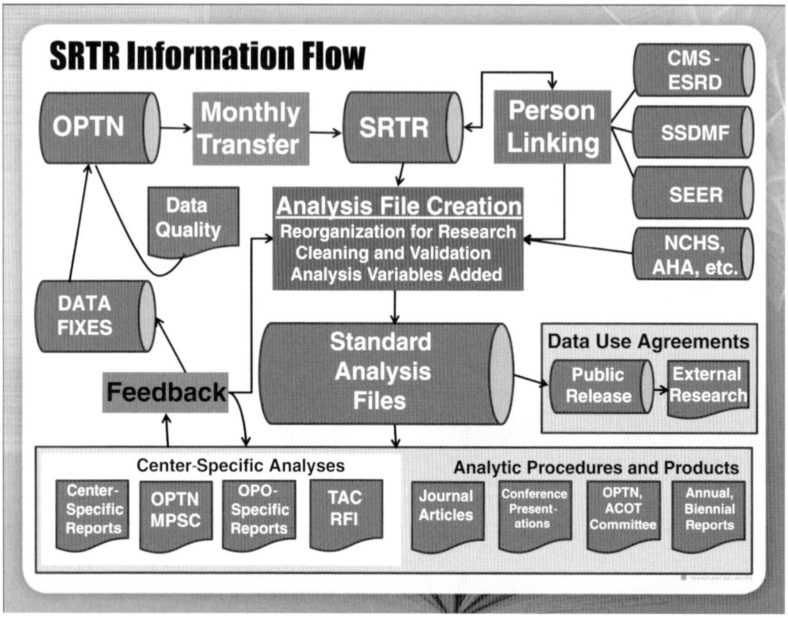

Figure 9.5 SRTR information flow.
Source: Scientific Registry of Transplant Recipients. *The SRTR Program-Specific Reporting Tools: Key Points.* http://www.srtr.org *(accessed January 7, 2014).*

July. Prior to the reports going public, in April and October, each transplant center has an opportunity to review their data, make corrections, and complete data submission for the next release. When the tables are finalized, transplant centers can provide comment as part of the publicly published report, giving the center an opportunity to explain unusual circumstances that are not evident in the report.

The published PSRs are a valuable resource for transplant centers, commercial insurance companies, CMS, and patients and families because they provide a wealth of statistical information, such as, the average time a patient spends on the center's waitlist before transplant, the organ specific center mortality rate (death on the waitlist), and survival rates for 1 month, 1 year and 3 years. Using a risk-adjusted model, the SRTR compares observed rates (the actual negative events that occur in a center) against what might be expected based on donor and recipient characteristics at all centers regionally and nationally. [13–15]. Risk adjustment is a statistical method that accounts for variation in characteristics of patient populations and/or geographical areas. Risk-adjusted survival data compare the center's own "expected" outcomes to regional and national outcomes and are supposed to provide an indication of whether the center is performing up to CMS standards [13]. "A center's (risk-adjusted) expected

1-year patient survival and 1-year graft survival will be compared to its observed 1-year patient survival and 1-year graft survival, based on the following non-compliance thresholds" [4]:

- Observed deaths or graft losses minus expected >3 (O-E > 0.3)
- Observed deaths or graft losses divided by expected >1.5 (O/E > 1.5)
- One-sided p <0.05 (statistical significance, not related to chance)

The biggest issue that most transplant centers have with the SRTR is that 1-year survival, the current benchmark for CMS recertification, is based on lagging data. (Note: It is anticipated that 3-year survival will soon be a CMS benchmark.) While the SRTR reports are published every 6 months, the cohorts of patients reported on were transplanted anywhere from 12 to 18 months before the publication date for 1-year outcomes. This methodology allows each patient at a center to have an opportunity to live for at least 1 year post-transplant and generally provides a large enough number of patients in the cohort to reflect a sufficiently sized sample. This requires a "2.5-year cohort ending 12–18 months before the report date, with some transplants occurring as long as 3.5 to 4 years before" [13], creating a significant lag time between the actual transplant and the report publication date. Many changes can take place in a transplant center and in the field of transplant science and care over 2 to 4 years.

Another concern about this methodology for evaluating transplant center performance is that differences in patient survival between centers as well as differences between the "expected" and the "observed" events at one center may be due to factors that are not readily apparent. Differences in a center's donor and recipient populations when compared to other regional centers may be significant enough to make comparison inadequate. For instance, one transplant center in a region may attract patients who require more complex care (e.g., ABO-incompatible transplants, or desensitization before transplant); these patients would have a higher degree of mortality risk that is not currently accounted for in the risk-adjustment model. Some Organ Procurement Organizations may draw from a Donor Service Area that is very urban or very rural. This difference in geography may account for significant differences in donor populations, making the donor pool more or less risky to the transplant center. There is also the possibility that differences in survival are due to chance or random variation.

Risk-adjustment models

Providing both observed and expected data allows for a better comparison among centers based on the patient populations they serve, although the factors included in the risk-adjustment models are not exhaustive and may not adequately represent patients or services provided by the center. The

SRTR uses several data sources for the model including the TRR form and the UNOS Deceased Donor Registration (DDR) form.

Some factors that are included in the SRTR risk-adjustment models are [13]

- recipient and donor demographic characteristics such as age, weight, and race;
- ABO compatibility;
- primary disease of the recipient;
- donor cause of death;
- ischemia time;
- previous transplant;
- if the recipient was on life support at time of transplant;
- Human Leukocyte Antigen (HLA) mismatch and Panel Reactive Antibodies (PRA) (KIDNEY);
- duration on dialysis (KIDNEY);
- creatinine (LIVER).

Each one of these factors has a "weighted coefficient," which gives it a greater or lesser amount of risk in the model. One month before the PSRs are published, the SRTR makes the risk-adjustment models available online to the center. The model provides information specific to that cohort about what factors were included in the model, as well as the positive or negative beta coefficient (factor weight) as well as the probability (p-value) that there is a real effect (not due to chance) related to this characteristic [13]. High risk conditions are represented by positive beta coefficients where as negative coefficients reference lower risk conditions. Not every factor about every patient can be included in a model, and this can also pose problems for a center. Factors such as recipient income, education, or health literacy are not included, neither are the recipient's nutritional status, smoking status, employment status, or all comorbidities [14]. If a center transplants more patients of a lower socioeconomic status, with low health literacy, and poor nutritional status, then the center's expected outcome may not accurately reflect the center's true risk, because these risk factors, which have been shown to increase survival risk, are not included in the current SRTR model. This discrepancy between expected and observed may cause the center to be flagged by CMS for non-compliance with outcomes. Figure 9.6 depicts a sample kidney risk-adjustment model; note that a patient with a diagnosis of hypertensive nephrosclerosis has a higher beta coefficient (0.0030) than a recipient with polycystic kidney disease (–0.3855), demonstrating hypertensive nephrosclerosis has a higher risk for mortality in this model [13]. The SRTR recognizes that their current approach of measuring center performance is not as robust in predicting performance as other

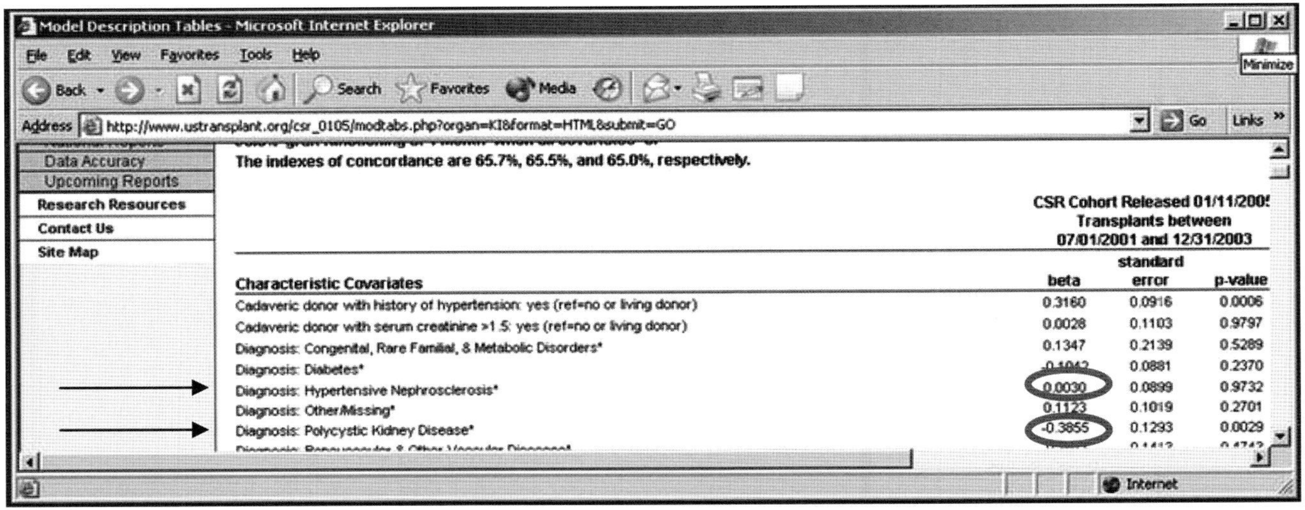

Figure 9.6 Example of a risk-adjustment model for kidney transplant.

Source: Scientific Registry of Transplant Recipients. *The SRTR Program-Specific Reporting Tools: Key Points.* http://www.srtr.org (*accessed January 7, 2014*).

methodologies. In particular, a Bayesian methodology has been identified as being superior in that it gives the probability that a center's performance does meet a certain standard [16]. The assumption is that basically all programs perform about average and that data must be overwhelmingly compelling to shift performance outside the statistical norm. This is a huge benefit for small-volume transplant programs where one death may result in being noncompliant with outcomes. The MPSC, CMS and the SRTR are in the process of evaluating this new model.

The benefits of retrospective and prospective analysis

Understanding the risk-adjustment models and the factors that are included or excluded in determining expected outcomes are important to understanding past performance, but these model worksheets can also be used to predict future performance and the individual risks for each candidate added to a center's waitlist. A transplant center can download their most recent SRTR risk tables, and keep a running spreadsheet of their recent recipients to assess one-year survival probability based on the current model. This practice may help to identify those patients who may be at higher risk for mortality. It is important to note here that risk-adjustment models do change—factors may be added or deleted over time, and factor weights may change as well. By using the SRTR risk adjustment models, the team can take a proactive approach to reducing morbidity and mortality. Examples of this would be, implementing a more stringent monitoring protocol to identify issues like rejection or infection earlier, or providing a post-transplant program of ongoing and frequent multidisciplinary support and education to increase self-care effectiveness and adherence.

The risk-adjustment spreadsheet can also be used as a predictive tool during the selection conference as part of the evaluation discussion. By adding a potential candidate to the cohort spreadsheet, the team can evaluate a specific patient's estimated one-year mortality risk using data scenarios for an average donor, a low-risk donor, or a high-risk donor. This is a good way to prospectively determine the amount of risk that each patient brings to transplant, to a possible patient cohort, and the amount of risk that may be taken in donor selection as organ offers occur. Many centers routinely use the SRTR risk-adjustment spreadsheets at the selection conference for exactly this purpose.

Another way a transplant center can use the predictive models is to determine how much risk a program can take over a period of time, i.e., tolerance for negative events. The SRTR cohorts roll forward in 6-month increments, from January 1 to June 30, and from July 1 to December 31. As each cohort rolls forward, the cohort is "set" for the time period and the volume of transplants that has taken place during that 6-month period. The more volume a transplant center does during the cohort period, the less impact each negative event has on the cohort, and vice versa. For instance, using an example of a transplant center that does 20 lung transplants a year, if the transplants are fairly evenly spread, for example, 10 transplants every 6 months, then the impact of one death in the cohort gives them roughly a 90% survival rate (1 negative event out of 10). But if the transplant center did 14 transplants in one 6-month period and only four the next, the tolerance of one negative event in each cohort is very different (92.8% survival, vs. 75%). In this example, if the expected survival was 84%, then the tolerance for the first cohort of 14 patients would be two negative events for an observed survival of 85.7%; there is zero tolerance for any negative event in the second cohort. Once a cohort is set in terms of the total number of patients, a transplant center can estimate the amount of risk they can withstand within the cohort and predict how many negative events they can "tolerate" before they are pushed over the "flagging" threshold. This type of assessment may allow a transplant center to consider small numbers of higher risk patients. In this highly regulated environment, a transplant center may be figuratively paying for the sins of the past, due to lagging reporting methodology. However, understanding future cohorts of patients is critically important because it will provide the roadmap for where you are going in real time under current circumstances, current staff, and current care practices and hopefully provide the transplant center with the knowledge needed to avoid future outcomes issues.

In addition to the survival statistics for patient and graft outcomes, the SRTR PSR's provide many other statistics such as waitlist mortality, transplant rate, and length of stay (LOS) post-transplant [13]. Waitlist mortality and transplant rate are two additional criteria along with survival outcomes that CMS uses to evaluate transplant centers [13].

The Transplant Administrator will spend a significant amount writing and implementing corrective action plans, and responding to CMS, OPTN, and commercial payers when outcomes or volumes are lower than expected. Being flagged twice by CMS in a 24 month period, will put the transplant center on the path to a contract for a Systems Improvement Agreement (SIA) with CMS to maintain center certification. During the SIA, the center will need to demonstrate that it has at least 0.5 full-time employee (FTE) dedicated to QAPI for the duration of the SIA. Understanding how to use the SRTR PSRs and risk-adjustment models is a critical skill. The transplant administrator should invest in developing a strong analytically capable QAPI team, by hiring personnel that can manage the data analysis and reporting needs that are mandated by CMS. Quality Analysts are becoming a de facto requirement for Transplant QAPI. These highly skilled team members are important for overall quality program management and managing ongoing outcomes analysis. In the absence of a quality analyst, the Transplant Administrator may be responsible for these activities. Given the labor-intensive and specialized knowledge required for a robust QAPI program, this is a resource that must be fully supported and funded. Establishing strong data management practices that support data integrity and accuracy, as well a strength in QAPI, are just as important to a center as the provision of excellent clinical care. Living and dying by the SRTR reporting is reality—your center's viability depends on it—continued Medicare certification and payment eligibility as well as commercial contracts are all rolled up tightly as measures of quality defined by volumes and clinical outcomes.

Data integrity

Though this whole chapter has been about data, we have yet to touch on data integrity, and it is not due to its lack of importance. In "computer speak," GIGO stands for Garbage In, Garbage Out, meaning if you put bad data into your computer system do not expect to get anything better out of it. Accuracy in the gathering, analysis, and reporting of data is critical, and error in any phase of data management can have immediate and/or long-term consequences. Some examples of data errors include:

- patient death due to incorrectly documenting a transplant candidate's ABO blood type (Sentinel Event);
- regulatory noncompliance caused by repeated data entry errors, for example, digit transposition in SSN, date of birth (DOB) (considered an administrative error on the UNOS Survey), or the creatinine level for a model for end-stage liver disease (MELD) score (rated as a clinical error on the UNOS survey);
- loss of commercial contracts caused by high SRTR "expected" values stemming from inadvertent overestimation of patient functional status on TRR forms.

These are just a few examples of how data integrity, or the lack of, can cause permanent and lasting harm to a transplant program. Whether transplant centers use transplant coordinators or dedicated data coordinators to enter data, it is important to provide training in accurate and standardized data entry to produce the most accurate statistical reflection of a program's outcomes. Unfortunately, there are also a number of ways that the system might be taken advantage of (intentionally or unintentionally). For instance, currently, if a center purposely omits patient data, e.g., race, this may provide the center an edge in their expected results because missing data may have a higher risk factorial than what the patient's actual race would provide. Suppose a center's patient's are all Caucasian, (the least risky racial status) and they omit race status on all patient reporting to UNOS. When their expected survival is calculated, the SRTR fills in an average risk factor for this patient's due to missing data, and by doing so, has just decreased the "expected survival" for this center, because the national data includes percentages of all other racial groups that carry higher risk. The center may benefit from this data omission. When data is missing, in some instances, the SRTR fills in the data using the national "average" for that data element. Let's use the previous example of beta co-efficients for ESRD diagnoses. If the diagnosis is missing for a patient with Polycystic Kidney Disease (PCKD), the SRTR will add an average co-efficient to the center's data set, which will likely be much higher than the PCKD weight, which carries fairly low risk. In this case, the center benefits from a lower expected survival, when compared to observed, for a patient that may not be high risk. It can also produce negative effects for a center. Suppose the center used the diagnosis of glomerular disease for all patients, to make data entry easy. This diagnosis is the co-efficient that all other diagnoses are compared to and carries a 0.0000 weight. But in this case, most of the center's patients have diabetes related ESRD. This center will be disadvantaged by suboptimal data management. The result will be that the center's expected outcomes will be much higher and may cause the center to have lower than expected outcomes, purely due to poor data management. While it is hoped that these types of data management concerns are not used intentionally by a center to create an undeserved advantage, the SRTR and the OPTN are aware of these possible situations, and are researching methods that will decrease this possible form of gaming.

It is imperative that the transplant administrator fully understand the importance of data integrity and accuracy and the impact data management has on a transplant center's ultimate success and viability. The transplant administrator must provide the leadership and resources to develop staff orientation and education plans that include data accuracy and integrity competencies in all processes and practices.

The burden for data management, analysis, and accountability on transplant centers is large and continues to grow. The Transplant Center must collect and report demographic and clinical data for their patients during all phases of transplant; these reported data are analyzed and translated into clinical outcomes; clinical outcomes drive regulatory compliance, upon which is critically hinged ongoing certification and commercial contracts, which is linked to the financial survival of the transplant center. Transplant administrators must understand the transplant workflow and data needs, to sufficiently address information management and knowledge generation. Transplant administrators must also be well-informed about tools to support staff in these areas.

As noted previously, despite more rapid adoption of EHR's in healthcare, most are not specifically built to handle the specialized data needs and workflows of the transplant center. Specialized transplant information systems (sometimes called niche systems) meet many transplant requirements for patient monitoring, analyzing clinical outcomes, performing research, and regulatory reporting, but may not fully (or at all), integrate with a certified EHR. Existing between these parallel electronic worlds, a transplant information system is deemed better than managing QAPI and outcomes using antiquated paper-based systems. Nevertheless, two systems will create multiple pain points for transplant staff, in terms of redundant medication and problem lists, duplicate documentation pathways, and physical silos of information.

Transplant programs that still rely on paper records and methods for data and information management will be increasingly disadvantaged in their ability to comply with routine regulatory and business requirements. They will be ineffective and inefficient in managing personnel and other resources, and may be insufficiently resourced to deliver the highest quality of patient care.

Effective transplant leaders must guide their programs in resource management, identifying and acquiring human resources and being highly involved in selecting hardware and software applications. They should identify and hire qualified personnel to manage electronic systems, ensure data integrity and accuracy, perform quality analysis, and generate valuable transplant information and knowledge from the system. Transplant leaders should also be actively involved in all opportunities for system selection, purchase, implementation, and evaluation and should be able to critically examine a system with both enterprise and transplant program requirements in mind. The investment in information technology is substantial, and having a business plan that provides compelling reasons to senior leaders for such a large investment is crucial.

References

1 Nelson R. Major theories supporting health care informatics. In: Englebardt SP, Neslon R, eds. *Health Care Informatics: An Interdisciplinary Approach*. Mosby, St. Louis; 2002:3–27.
2 Keck BM, Daily OP. Data requirements of OPTN members. In Phillips MG, ed. *UNOS Organ Procurement, Preservation and Distribution in Transplantation*. 2nd ed. Richmond: UNOS; 1996:311–345.
3 United Network for Organ Sharing. *History of Database*. http://www.unos.org/donation/index.php?topic=history_of_database. Accessed September 10, 2012.
4 Centers for Medicare & Medicaid Services (CMS). Conditions for Coverage (CfCs) & Conditions of Participations (CoPs)–Transplant Centers. http://www.cms.gov/Reg

ulations-and-Guidance/Legislation/CFCsAndCoPs/transplantcenters.html. Accessed November 17, 2012.

5 Tang PC, McDonald CJ. Computer-based patient-record systems. In: Shortliffe EH, Cimino JJ, eds. *Biomedical Informatics; Computer Applications in Health Care and Biomedicine*. 3rd ed. New York: Springer; 2006:335–370.

6 Sackett KM, Erdley WS. The history of health care informatics. In: Englebardt SP, Nelson R, eds. *Health Care Informatics: an interdisciplinary approach*. Mosby, St. Louis; 2002:3–27.

7 Thede LQ. Understanding databases. In: Englebardt SP, Nelson R. eds. *Health Care Informatics: An Interdisciplinary Approach*. Mosby, St. Louis; 2002:55–80.

8 Markus BH, Mitchell S, Gordon RD, Gillauist B, Tzakis AG, Starzl TE. TIMY-a center-oriented transplant information. *Transplant Proc*. 1988;20(1)1, Suppl. 1:385–390.

9 Kearns LE. 2008Patient Alerts—A Vehicle to Identify a Vocabulary. Unpublished Paper.

10 U.S. Department of Health & Human Services. HITECH Act Enforcement Interim Final Rule http://www.hhs.gov/ocr/privacy/hipaa/administrative/enforcementrule/hitechenforcementifr.html. Accessed August 31, 2012.

11 The HITECH Act. Accessed on January 28, 2011, at http://www.gpo.gov/fdsys/pkg/PLAW-111publ5/pdf/PLAW-111publ5.pdf. Accessed August 31, 2012.

12 Marion J. Cardiovascular Information Systems - Is CVIS relevant in an ARRA/meaningful use world? Healthcare Informatics. January 2012 3, p. 23–27.

13 Scientific Registry of Transplant Recipients. The SRTR Program-Specific Reporting Tools: Key Points. http://www.srtr.org/csr/current/tech_notes.aspx. Aaccessed January 7, 2014.

14 Schold JD, Arrington CJ, Levine G. Significant alternations in reported clinical practice associated with increased oversight of organ transplant center performance. *Prog Transplant*. 2011;20:279–287.

15 Schold JD. You Don't Know What You Don't Know: Forecasting SRTR Transplant Center Reports. UNOS Transplant Management Forum, April, 2012.

16 Under Construction: Transplant Center Award Criteria. Donation and Transplantation Community of Practice (DTCP). http://healthcarecommunities.org/DTCP/. July 27, 2010. Transplant Webinar. Accessed December 8, 2012.

CHAPTER 10
Strategy and Marketing

Lisa Norris
Transplant Leadership Institute LLC, San Antonio, TX, USA

Strategic planning

A strategic plan determines the overall course the business will take in the future. Successful transplant programs must devote time and energy in developing and crafting a strategic plan in order to ensure long-term success. This is particularly important in the new reality of a highly regulated and unpredictable healthcare environment where strategy needs to be more adaptable and flexible. Creating an achievable and dynamic strategic plan requires a data-driven methodology that is focused on outcomes and measurability and adjusting as necessary. Major stakeholders (physicians, surgeons, senior leaders, transplant administrator) in the program must be a part of the planning process in addition to staff. Inclusion of the entire team in the process creates buy-in and alignment toward goals.

Planning begins with developing a mission and vision which serves as a foundation for future success and should align with the larger organization's mission and vision. Often mission and vision statements are mistakenly interchanged, however, they are quite separate and have a different focus. The mission statement is a concise statement describing the program and its goal, whereas the vision statement describes what the program desires to be in the future.

Examples of Mission and Vision Statements

Mission statements

- The Department of Organ Transplantation is a group of highly qualified and compassionate professionals who pride themselves in providing outstanding care for both patients and families. We respect individuals for their contribution; support professional and personal development; and join together compassion with medicine in meeting the spiritual, social and physical needs of patients and their families.

Transplant Administration, First Edition. Edited by Lisa Norris.

Companion website: www.wiley.com/go/norris/transplantadmin

- Our mission is to provide kidney transplantation to the patients and families we serve through a multi-disciplinary approach to care creating a high standard of care in a safe and supportive environment.
- The transplant center's mission is to
  - provide outstanding multi-disciplinary and integrated clinical care throughout the entire continuum of care from end-stage organ disease through post transplant care;
  - support basic science in the field of transplantation and foster innovation and new scientific discoveries;
  - mentor future physician and scientific leaders in transplantation;
  - Build a robust referral base to sustain operations;
  - Be a strong participant in the development of public policy in the field of organ donation and transplantation.

Vision statements

- By 2015, the transplant institute will be nationally recognized as one of the top 10 transplant programs in the United States where patients want to come for outstanding care and experience, the very best surgeons, physicians and healthcare professionals want to practice.
- Our vision is to be the trusted leader in transplant care and advancing the health of our patients.
- To become nationally recognized for outcomes, volumes, patient satisfaction, and best value and to position the transplant institute as having the best state-of-the-art, compassionate care.
- The vision of the transplant institute is to be the program of choice for state-of-the-art care, and innovative research, with a dedication to excellence in all that we do.

Other principal components of the strategic plan are

- environmental assessment;
- identification of your program's strengths, weaknesses, opportunities, and threats (SWOT);
- development of specific goals within a 3–5-year time span;
- development of an action plan to obtain the desired goals;
- performance monitoring by identifying milestones.

Collecting data concerning the external and internal environment is important to the overall planning process. Examples of data that should be collected are given in Table 10.1. Once key data have been collected, reviewed, and discussed, a SWOT analysis should be performed. The SWOT analysis begins by assessing the internal strengths and weaknesses of the program which are identified by internal program review. Opportunities and threats are external to the program and should be identified after review of the data collected on competitors and the overall external environment [1].

- Strengths: characteristics of the program that give it an advantage
- Weaknesses: limitations of the program which serve as a disadvantage

Table 10.1 Data collection for strategic planning

Internal data such as volume and referrals
Population growth
Area demographics
Disease prevalence and projected prevalence
Transplants per million
Referral patterns
Market share of area transplant programs
Competitor survival statistics
Competitor transplant volume by organ and type
Insurance contracts
Donation service area statistics

- Opportunities: *external* chances to improve or expand
- Threats: *external* elements in the environment that could jeopardize the program or its growth

Questions to ask when examining strengths and weaknesses:

- Who are our customers?
- Who are our competitors? Are they local, regional, national?
- What is the economic environment and how will that affect the program?
- What new technology is available and will that be an opportunity?
- What changes are there in the regulatory environment?
- What are our limiting factors? Donors? Staff? Resources?
- Does the program have internal capacity for growth?

An example of a transplant-specific SWOT analysis can be found in Table 10.2. The goals that are set for the program should be based on the program's vision statement. For example, if the vision is to be the region's transplant program of choice, possible goals might include increasing referrals, expansion of services, and improving patient satisfaction. A financial plan may or may not be a part of the planning process, but knowing the resources needed to execute the plan should be accomplished in order to move the strategy forward. Specifying how goals will be measured along with timelines and those who are responsible for executing the plan are important factors to be included. Regular meetings with key stakeholders to keep the plan on track should be scheduled. Lastly, progress toward achieving goals must be communicated to all members of the transplant team on a periodic basis. Several examples of strategic planning tools are found in Tables 10.3 and 10.4. Although similar, these tools both highlight the important points to keep in mind when formulating a detailed strategic plan.

Table 10.2 Example of kidney transplant SWOT

Strengths • Strong referral base • Good public relations exposure over past few years • Outreach clinics • Comprehensive program: includes pediatrics and adults • OR and bed capacity available for expansion • Financially viable	**Weaknesses** • Significant delays in donor and recipient evaluations • Critical pathways process not present on unit • Inexperienced coordinators • Nephrology/transplant not optimizing their relationship; lack integrated, multi-disciplinary team • Need to improve communications with referring physicians • Limited information systems/database
Opportunities • New modalities such as steroid-free protocol and desensitization • Paired donation • CME courses for referring physicians • Create relationships with dialysis clinics	**Threats** • Staff retention • RN shortage • Four renal transplant programs in city • Aggressive reimbursement by payers • Poor performing OPO • Healthcare reform • Physician reimbursement

Marketing

A marketing plan is a key component of the strategic plan in that it strengthens the linkages between the environment and the business or program. It should support the mission of the hospital and transplant program and assist in determining where marketing resources can be channeled in order to achieve the goals of the program. Marketing is about creating, communicating, delivering, and exchanging offerings that have value for customers, whether the customers are patients, referring physicians, or collaborating organizations [2]. There are more than 5700 hospitals and approximately 250 transplant centers in the United States, many of which are in metropolitan areas [3, 4]. Competition is fierce to attract both patients and referrals. Marketing one's organization is crucial in today's competitive environment not to so much to drive demand but to differentiate one program from another. The components of a good transplant marketing plan consist of four main areas: identifying the target market, market research, branding, and communication to customers.

Market research/target markets

The first question to be asked in order to formulate a marketing plan is who is our customer? Customers can be grouped into segments with similar needs or target markets. For a transplant program, the main target markets

Table 10.3 Strategic business plan: implementation and monitoring plan

Implementation	Responsible person/s	Monitoring	Resources needed	Time lines
Overall program objective: *Increase patients referred, patient access to services, and transplant volumes.*				
Abdominal transplantation program expansion				
1. Gain consensus on direction of program and intention to support and sustain long-term growth	Jones	Strategic plan reviewed by all key decision-makers. Changes to plan as required obtaining agreement and allowing input of stakeholders. Commitment to funding and implementation of strategic plan		December 2011
2. Redesign of protocols, policies, and procedures to reflect new leadership input and to achieve transplant goals	Jones, Smith, and Davis	Policies updated Inpatient drug costs Number of waitlisted patients Number of living donor transplants Number of deceased donor transplants Number for DCD organs procured at own facility Percentage of ECD and DCD transplants Waiting time Transplantation rate Patent and graft survival Organ acceptance rate		Ongoing

(continued)

Table 10.3 (*Continued*)

Implementation	Responsible person/s	Monitoring	Resources needed	Time lines
3. Living donor paired exchange program; develop cooperative agreement with other transplant hospitals for participation; develop policy for procedure; determine manpower and impact of workload logistics; review patients who were turned down due to incompatibility with living donors; dedicate staff to manage	Smith	Cooperative agreement in place Policies developed First exchange	Availability of plasmaphresis, OR capacity to accommodate two LD transplants per week	July 2011
4. Provide hotel and access to outpatient services to promote early discharge	Davis	Length of stay Average charges	Completion of transplant guest house	August 2011
5. Implement high PRA reduction protocol to improve transplantation opportunities for highly sensitized patients; obtain state-level efforts to get local Medicare FI to pay for therapy	Smith and Jones	Number of patients entered into new protocol Number of transplants performed using new protocol Payment for protocol State and local policy change	Availability of plasmaphresis	July 2011
6. Design space to accommodate efficient operations	Harris	Adequate space for staff, storage, and meetings	Redesign of transplant office space which will include $25,000 for office cubicles and furniture	October 2011
7. Decrease ICU days	Wood	ICU days per case Cost per case	Improve education of nurses in unit, dedicated transplant unit with monitoring	January 2012

Vascular access surgery/expansion of services			
1. Perform access placement before dialysis is required	Wood	Number of predialysis patients receive access	November 2012
2. Evaluation of potential to perform access cases at lower cost facility than hospital based	Wood	Team in place to evaluate possibilities and physician practice plan allows physicians to own and operate	October 2012
Other transplant services			
1. Enhance pediatric transplant program	Jones	Volume Survival	January 2013
2. Enhance pancreas transplantation	Davis	Patients evaluated Patients listed Patients transplanted	January 2013
National recognition			
1. Active membership participation and presentations in national and international professional organizations	Harris	Number of presentations, and participation in organizations	January 2013
2. Support market-based standards for staff education, credentialing, and certification	Jones	Standards incorporated into job descriptions and supported Salaries benchmarked internally and externally	October 2013
3. Publication in professional journals	Davis	Number of publications	Ongoing
4. Comparison of patient and family satisfaction scores to internal and external benchmarks	Smith	Internal scores External benchmarking scores	August 2013

(*continued*)

Table 10.3 *(Continued)*

Implementation	Responsible person/s	Monitoring	Time lines
Transplantation differentiation of services from competition			
1. Contact with referring physicians and dialysis centers at the time of financial approval, time of listing, and time of transplant	Baker	Contacts completed	January 2013
2. Monitoring utilization of services, following established protocols and maximizing use of alternative levels of care	Holly	LOS, ICU days, cost of drugs	September 2013 and ongoing
3. Improved workup time, management of waitlist, contact with patients on waitlist and introduction of coordinator who will be following the patient	Harris	Evaluation time frames Patient contacts Patient on status 7 decreased	October 2013

Table 10.4 Strategic plan implementation grid

			Proposed solution						
Priority	Category	Issue/Opportunity	Proposed solution	Who	How	Benchmarking support	Cost vl	Benefit	Timing
Liver									
1	Organ access	Next exporter of organs	Evaluate program decision-making process on organ selection	Transplant surgeons	Consensus on use of dcd, ecd organs		Low	High	Near term
2	Patient mix	Optimize patient mix; believe opportunity for growing liver cancer transplants	Engage oncologists on option of liver transplant, internally and externally	Hepatologists/Txp Surgeons	Partner with oncology, liver ablation/resection		Low	High	Med term
3	Targeted growth	Believe additional opportunity to do clinics in untapped markets	Set up satellites in identified locations	Physician teams (with outreach support?)	Complete geo analysis, assess physician bandwidth requirements, identify locations to house satellite efforts	Known models of flying hep-atologists to outreach locations	Med	High	Near term

(continued)

Table 10.4 *(Continued)*

Priority	Category	Issue/Opportunity	Proposed solution			Benchmarking support	Cost lvl	Benefit	Timing
			Proposed solution	Who	How				
4	Marketing	Currently not recognized as biggest, best, most comprehensive institution for liver care	Increase marketing efforts—direct to patient, with referral community, with peer groups	Add a marketing resource to txp center	Peer marketing, TBD		High	High	Near term
5	Resources—personnel	Retention of key physicians problematic; also defecting to regional competition	Develop incentives to attract and retain top talent to maintain program's position of strength	Hospital leadership must agree to incentives	Base salary + bonus based on some agreed measure of productivity		High	High	Med term
6	Resources—institution	Lack of dedicated ICU beds alienates referring MDs	Make beds available to transplant (priority)	Hospital leadership must agree to this			High	High	Near term
7	Resources—institution	OR congestion limits capacity for multiple cases/rapid turnover	Require policy for OR access given timing requirements of transplant	Hospital operations (COO) with surgeon buy-in required	Ensure all ORs optimized; then define principles driving transplant prioritization; roll-out prioritization policy (TBD)		High	High	Near term

are: the primary target market consisting of patients, referring physicians, and managed care organizations; the secondary target market comprising organizations that are professional, disease state or regulatory in nature (such as the organ procurement organization, UNOS, and National Kidney Foundation); the tertiary target market which is the program's own hospital and/or health system—it is surprising that many organizations are unaware of the services and accomplishments of their very own transplant program.

Understanding the target markets and the needs of customers is also important. Although pertinent data may have been gathered as part of the strategic planning process, information on customer preferences and satisfaction can be derived from patient focus groups, patient satisfaction surveys, and physician surveys. The data generated from these surveys will provide additional insight into the mind of the customer. If the transplant program does not have a formal process for gathering this type of information, an easy online survey tool, SurveyMonkey, is quite helpful [5].

Branding

Building the image and reputation of the transplant program is the function of branding. The cornerstone of the marketing plan should be the brand of the program which should shape the perceptions and touch the emotions of the customer. A brand is the result of what the organization is, says, and does as it interfaces with patients, physicians, employees, vendors, the community—and the emotional feelings that are engendered by that interaction. Image advertising and promotion are especially effective in increasing brand recognition to customers. It usually takes the form of a slogan or message which conveys name, mission, proficiency, supportiveness, or technological expertise. "We're Here For Life," "Leading, Teaching, Caring," and "Serious Medicine—Extraordinary Care"—all are examples of messages (taken from existing institutions) that convey a feeling which increases awareness and influences choice. However, branding goes beyond marketing—it also is conveyed by the friendliness of staff, the look and feel of your clinics, the cleanliness of the facility, and many other aspects of the program. In other words, the message of image promotion must be matched by the customer experience for believability to occur.

Communication to customers

Communication to customers encompasses a vast array of marketing activities and should be focused both externally and internally to the organization or transplant program. Examples of activities are

- website development, both internet and intranet;
- speeches to professional organizations; receptions; seminars, patient celebrations; grand rounds;

- physician interviews on television and radio talk shows;
- books, journal articles, abstracts;
- mainstream advertising;
- public and community relations;
- charity sponsorships;
- special events;
- social media, blogs, and social networks.

Internet and intranet presence

First and foremost, a transplant program should have an internet presence via a webpage which is typically a page within the website of the overall organization. Approximately 78.3% of the US population uses the internet and it is the primary way a patient or potential patient acquires information about any service or business [6]. A website should be professional and convey outcomes, staff credentials, and other programmatic information that will attract potential patients. Including patient testimonials is also powerful in communicating the clinical competence, ease, and friendliness of the program. A webpage should be updated often and should also be optimized for the various search engines so that patients can easily find your program. It is also important to measure the number of visits to your website in order to measure its effectiveness. A wonderful free tool is Google Analytics which will provide a number of valuable pieces of information: number of visitors, pages visited most often, keywords used for search (good for search engine optimization), traffic sources, and browser usage reports.

Internally, the transplant program should also have an intranet presence so that those within the organization become aware of the transplant enterprise and the value to the overall organization. The program should use this platform to promote accomplishments, celebrations, educational activities, and special events.

Mainstream advertising

Although we have entered the age of the electronic media and the internet, traditional advertising still plays a role in marketing and creating customer awareness. Because transplant is a niche specialty, the use of broad-based advertising media is not very cost-effective. Some of the common modes of advertising are

- Billboards: These reach more people per dollar than any other media but are overall expensive and used mainly by hospitals to increase awareness.
- Radio: Reaches a significant number of people and can be targeted; however, is also a costly form of advertising.

- Television: Very expensive and so used by hospitals to increase demand and awareness.
- Newspapers and magazines: Can target by readership and circulation; however, very expensive and is losing share to social media.
- Direct mail: Highly targeted mode of advertising; however, is also very costly to produce and mail.
- Flyers/brochures: Highly targeted and used to communicate information about the transplant program or new technologies.
- Annual reports: Also used to reach a specific audience. Expensive but an impressive method to communicate the effectiveness of the overall transplant program, physician competencies, successes, research, outreach, and poignant patient stories.

Public relations

One of the most highly effective and lowest cost marketing alternatives is public relations. There is an old adage "advertising is paid for, publicity is prayed for." Both advertising and public relations are important; however, the advantages of public relations are that it basically is at no cost and comes from independent media which patients and other customers view as impartial and credible. Public relations encompass activities such as public appearances by caregivers, news releases, patient stories, events, celebrations, and interviews. Examples of newsworthy items are successful or unique patient stories, awards, and recognition, and novel surgical techniques or therapies. It is important for the transplant program to partner with their hospital's public relations department and to keep them informed about newsworthy items and to collaborate on developing press releases.

Social media

Social media has become a wildly popular mode of marketing in recent years. According to the 2012 Social Media Marketing Industry Report, 85% of marketers reported that social media increased their business exposure and increased traffic to the company website (69%) [7]. Social media should be integrated into the program's overall marketing plan to augment existing strategies. So what exactly is social media? This form of marketing is really a technique which utilizes various social media services in order to build relationships, develop a loyal following, and to promote thought leadership. It is low cost, however it is time intensive. This encompasses

- Blogs: Websites which have changing content that allow readers to post their own viewpoints or opinions
- Social networking sites: Facebook, Twitter, and others
- Social media sites: Sites where video, photographs, and audio can be posted: YouTube, Flickr, Podcast alley, Pinterest

These sites can be thought of as an electronic "word of mouth." Consumers of healthcare are increasingly turning to these sites to gather information and share experiences. In fact, one survey of consumers of hospital social media and the influence of choice found:

- Fifty-seven percent of consumers indicated that a hospital's social media offerings would have a great influence on their use of that hospital's services.
- Twenty-five percent of consumers said they would probably visit a hospital's social media site in the future.
- Eighty-one percent of consumers said that a strong social media presence made them feel that a hospital's services were cutting edge [8].

The social media experience of the Methodist Healthcare System in Houston is found in the following case study. This case study highlights how social media can be a powerful tool to augment the patient experience and to share a hospital's culture. It has direct applicability to a transplant program which is really just a subset of the larger organization. Most transplant programs have developed separate sites on Facebook, however they require further enhancement. Using the hospital's platform for highlighting the transplant program may provide the best exposure.

Case study: Social Media Case Study

In 2009, the Methodist Hospital System in Houston, Texas, started on their journey into the world of social media. They began with Facebook to highlight their hospital and their services. The first posts to their site were videos from TV commercials; however, they then added content related to patient events and activities [1]. The strategy was to stimulate conversation by inviting patients, families, and employees to talk about the hospital. Posts provided health information to patients and also promoted the hospital with information about honors and rankings. Concurrently, the hospital also developed the use of Twitter, Blogs, and YouTube platforms. Twitter was used primarily to point consumers to the Methodist YouTube and Facebook sites [1]. Subsequently, Methodist developed a social media policy to guide personnel on posting guidelines and developed a social media strategy that focused on community outreach, brand awareness, customer service, education, public relations, crisis communications, and recruitment [1]. The hospital charged the Department of Public Relations with managing their social media and developing content. In fact, they tweet at least 2–3 times per day and according to Clare Rose, VP of Operations, "two thirds of the tweets are health news and about one-third are hospital promotions." [2]

In the future, the challenge will be to quantify the effectiveness of these platforms. However, today, Methodist has more than 4000 followers on Twitter and have realized a substantial increase in referrals overall [1].

References

1 Angell D, Rose C. Conversations with the community: the Methodist Hospital System's experience with social media. *Front Health Serv Manag.* 2012;28(2):15–21.

2 Squazzo J. Best practices for applying social media in healthcare. *Healthc Exec.* 2010;25(3):35–39.

References

1 Giacoma T. Fundamentals of successful transplant administration (Chapter 27). In: Lapointe D, Ohler L, Rudow T, eds. *A Clinician's Guide to Donation and Transplantation.* New York: Applied Measurement Professionals, Inc; 2006:3–4.

2 AHA Hospital Statistics 2012. American Hospital Association. http://www.aha.org/research/rc/stat-studies/fast-facts.shtml. Accessed October 14, 2013.

3 American Marketing Association. http://www.marketingpower.com/AboutAMA/Pages/DefinitionofMarketing.aspx. Accessed October 14, 2013.

4 HRSA Organ Procurement and Transplantation Network. http://optn.transplant.hrsa.gov/members/. Accessed October 14, 2013.

5 SurveyMonkey. www.surveymonkey.com. Accessed October 14, 2013.

6 Internet World Stats. http://www.internetworldstats.com/stats14.htm. Accessed October 14, 2013.

7 Stelzner M. Social media marketing industry report. *Soc Media Exam.* 2012 April 2012.

8 Beach-Thielst B. Social media: ubiquitous community and patient engagement. *Front Health Serv Manage.* 2012;28(2):3–14.

CHAPTER 11

Managing and Leading the Transplant Enterprise

Lisa Norris
Transplant Leadership Institute LLC, San Antonio, TX, USA

Previous chapters have illustrated that the transplant enterprise has inherent complexity and that there are many knowledge areas to master. This challenging and highly specialized enterprise demands extraordinary leadership and robust management in order to be successful. This chapter is really a call to action. The field of transplantation must develop leadership and formulate a plan on how to transition the next generation—the survival of the field depends on it.

Leadership and management are not necessarily the same. The late Stephen Covey said "Management is efficiency in climbing the ladder of success; leadership determines whether the ladder is leaning against the right wall" [1]. Indeed, leadership and management are two different, yet complimentary functions which are necessary for a well-run organization. Leadership, contrary to popular belief, is not about being charismatic or visionary (although it is an added plus), but is really the ability to cope with organizational and external change. Whereas, management is the ability to deal with complexity [2]. So how specifically are they different?

- Management
  - Planning and creating a budget
  - Organizing and staffing
  - Controlling and problem-solving
  - Taking complex systems and making them run efficiently and effectively
- Leadership
  - Communicating and setting direction
  - Motivating staff
  - Aligning people and developing relationships [3]

The widely held belief is that leaders are born not made. There may some truth to that statement, since some individuals do possess inherent

Transplant Administration, First Edition. Edited by Lisa Norris.

Companion website: www.wiley.com/go/norris/transplantadmin

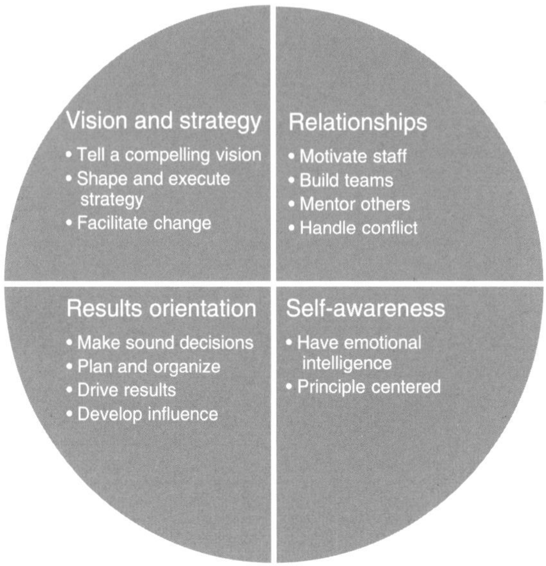

Figure 11.1 Leadership competencies
Source: Data from Gebelein SH, Nelson-Neuhaus KJ, Skube CJ, et al. *Successful Manager's Handbook*. 7th ed. Minneapolis, MN: Personal Decisions International; 2004:158.

leadership ability; however, leadership can also be learned and developed. So how can a person develop both skill sets? Michael Watkins in his recent article *How Managers Become Leaders* wrote, "They must learn to move from specialist to generalist, analyst to integrator, tactician to strategist, bricklayer to architect, problem solver to agenda setter, warrior to diplomat, and supporting cast member to lead role." According to Watkins, an individual must move through these seven seismic shifts in order to make the transition [4]. One transplant surgeon recently remarked that physicians and surgeons went to medical school, trained in residencies and fellowships, and then went into clinical practice—nothing really prepared them to lead a transplant enterprise. Many pursue an executive MBA, however, leadership and management skills are competencies not taught in the classroom. It is a process—a journey that one takes as experiences build upon another and self-awareness develops. Figure 11.1 depicts a leadership wheel with the various competencies and skills categorized and highlighted. The wheel highlights four dimensions of good leadership: self-awareness, relationships, vision and strategy, and results orientation. Each dimension is then further divided into those competencies that are essential to becoming an outstanding leader. Each one is described in detail below.

Self-awareness

- Become self-aware. Great leaders are able to assess their own strengths and weaknesses. They can view themselves in an objective manner and understand their motivations and emotions. They are open to receiving feedback and are willing to change course if valid and needed. Participation in a 360 degree evaluation is an excellent method to gather anonymous feedback from colleagues, superiors, and direct reports. It is a good way to find out how you are viewed by others and what changes are needed to improve performance. A free 360-degree tool is available online at www.reactive360.com/quick360.html. In addition, there are other tools (many free and online) such as Myers-Briggs, Johari Window, and DiSC tests that can assist in understanding personality and cognitive styles.

  Knowing your leadership style also can be very beneficial and there are many tools on the internet to assess one's style. The author Daniel Goleman identified six leadership styles in his book *Primal Leadership*: democratic, affiliative, pace-setter, visionary, coaching, and commanding [5]. Most individuals have a predominant style while using the other styles depending on the situation (also known as situational leadership). This flexibility is important in dealing with groups of diverse individuals with diverse needs similar to those found in multi-disciplinary teams. Goleman found that the more flexible a leader's style, the better the work environment and performance of the team. He also found that the more pace-setting and commanding the style, the more the team experienced burnout which resulted in high staff turnover [6]. The case study at the end of this section illustrates this point.

  Unfortunately, sometimes the culture of the organization and/or team is not a fit with a leader's style—this is a situation where coaching or mentoring might be beneficial. If all else fails, a parting of ways might be in everyone's best interest.
- Develop emotional intelligence. Emotional intelligence can be defined as the ability to manage emotions in order to excel in life and career. It can affect your mental and physical health, your personal life, and your career [7]. Negative emotions such as anger, disappointment, and grief from both the personal and professional sides of life can spill over onto other members of the team whether one realizes it or not. Thus, learning to respond professionally during emotional or stressful conditions is best for the team.
- Be principle-centered. The late Stephen Covey wrote an entire book on this subject entitled *Principle-Centered Leadership*. Principles are the natural laws of human nature or the human condition such as integrity,

fairness, honesty, justice, and trust [8]. Great leaders have at the core of their being these principles and tap into these principles as they interact with others. They lead by example and model exemplary behavior.

Case study

Hospital XYZ is a large academic medical center with a multi-organ transplant program located in a highly competitive urban area. Hospital XYZ's primary goal in 2003 was to achieve continued rapid growth and dominate the local market. Competition was fierce among the local transplant programs and the need to maintain volume was paramount. Staff described the program as chaotic with little emphasis on quality due to the emphasis on the volume of transplants. Burnout was widespread among the coordinators and morale was at an all-time low. Also noted were conflicting priorities among physicians, lack of regular communication from leadership, and inefficient work processes. The physician leader of the program was a true pace-setter: too involved in the day-to-day activities and driving the staff to achieve and work harder.

In early 2006, the program recruited a strong administrator who could organize and provide direction to the administrative, operations, and business needs of the program. The first order of business for the new administrator was to put into place clear and explicit work processes which included a redesign of the clinic flow, regular staff meetings, and a clear orientation program for all staff. Staffing levels were also addressed and schedules were changed to allow for more work–life balance. Clinical managers were hired to provide oversight for the clinical staff and to create more infrastructure. As these changes were put into place, the physician director also began his own transformation. He began to clearly define the program vision and motivated people to move in the same direction. He took a step back and began to temper his pace-setting nature. He also worked hard to form a strong partnership with the transplant administrator. Improvement began to be seen incrementally. Slowly, the program began to become more organized, and less chaotic. Staff morale improved and the program grew at a fast, yet measured pace. Four years later, the program was one of the largest in the United States with outstanding outcomes, and a stable staff. The moderation of a pace-setting leadership style along with the establishment of a partnership between the transplant administrator and the physician leader were the key elements of success in the turnaround of this transplant program.

Relationships

- Motivate staff. Leaders motivate staff by providing ways they can meet their needs while meeting organizational objectives. They are inspirational, self-assured, and radiate energy. They know that people are different and that they are motivated by different factors: money, title, achievement, and challenge—and they adjust accordingly. Some practical ways to motivate staff include matching the right person to the right job to ensure fit, ensure that performance evaluation measures adequately reflect the current task, involve staff in decision-making and important projects. Lastly, incorporate reward and recognition into the workplace and link it to meeting organizational goals. Rewards need not be costly—praise, credit, notes of appreciation, and celebrations all reinforce and motivate staff in the right direction.

- Build teams. Great leaders can identify talented individuals and assemble them into high-performing teams. Teams may come together for a short-term project or assignment or form for the long-term goals. Leading-edge transplant programs are those with self-directed work-teams: they solve problems, make day-to-day decisions, know their roles within the team, and reinvent and retool if the need arises. Effective leaders empower team members, and they facilitate, challenge, and support them. They value diversity of the team because they realize that different viewpoints and contributions strengthen the team and maximize creativity. They also ensure that the team has adequate resources in order to do the necessary work.
- Mentor others. Leaders develop a pipeline of talent who can assume more responsibility and can develop into future leaders. More will be said about this later in the chapter, however, mentoring can be individual or team based. In either case, the leader should share experiences, coach, offer encouragement, and point individuals in the right direction.
- Deal with conflict effectively. Conflict will inevitably arise in organizations, so the ability to deal with it head-on without fear is the key to influence and effectiveness. What is your reaction to conflict? Is it win-win, win-lose, or do you avoid conflict altogether? Obviously, a win-win style is the best option. Listen to both sides, get to the root of the problem, and then negotiate with both sides a workable solution. A win-lose style results in one party getting what they want at the expense of the other. Ignoring conflict is easiest, however, has equally poor outcomes. Warning signs of conflict aversion are delaying key decisions, making excessive compromises, telling people what they want to hear, discouraging opposing ideas, and delegating difficult situations to subordinates [9]. This behavior ultimately erodes trust and results in a dysfunctional organization. Be open to possibilities and tell the truth with tact and diplomacy and, if necessary, agree to disagree.

Vision and strategy

- Develop visioning. Being able to articulate a vision and energizing others in actualizing the vision is an important skill to develop. Visioning is about being able to look into the future and seeing where the organization or program must go in order to succeed. It involves combination of intuition, the ability to look at the big picture, and awareness of the developments in the external environment. In most transplant programs, the leader guides the team toward a shared vision. Once the vision has been determined, a leader must communicate a clear and consistent message in order to hardwire this into the team's culture [10]. The next step is to bring the vision into fruition. This is accomplished by setting goals, procedures, action plans, and other tools to move the team toward realizing the vision.

- Be strategic. A leader must be able to lead the organization through a process that will bring new ideas to the table and be innovative and entrepreneurial. They must be able to continually optimize strategies that challenge the organization's comfort zone and confront the reality of the need to do some things differently especially in this era of rapid change in healthcare. They must always be aware of the environment and the competition. In addition, a leader must be skilled in communicating mission and strategy.
- Facilitate change. Change is an ever-present fact in the world of transplantation, so it is important for a leader to be able to challenge the status quo and assist staff in accepting change. Building support for change among employees, patients, and other stakeholders is key prior to any action and it involves "selling" the benefit of the change. While the management team may want to drive change, staff often feels threatened by change and worry about their job security. Staff typically moves through three stages similar to that of grief: first is the letting go off the old and there may be anger, depression, and resistance; second is finding clarity amid the confusion and gaining acceptance; and third is the adoption of new ways and accepting the change. Managing change successfully requires initiating, communicating, and acquiring feedback of staff and involving staff along the way.

Results orientation

- Employ sound decision-making. This involves assessing options and risks, consulting people and taking their views and ideas into account, and gathering data and information. Be knowledgeable about financial statements, budgets, regulatory issues, and changes in the field. Analyze all available information and data. Weigh the alternatives taking into account how each alternative will affect others, organizational priorities, and the downstream consequences. Other factors to consider are cost, budget, legality, resources, and staffing. Select the best alternative and realize that there is usually no clear "right" decision. At times, the

Table 11.1 Decision matrix

Criteria	Database A	Database B	Database C	Database D
Data can be uploaded to UNOS	5	5	5	5
Labs and hospital EMR can be interfaced with database	4	2	5	5
Capital cost	5	2	1	1
Yearly maintenance cost	4	3	2	1
Ease of use	3	3	4	4
Has mobile phone feature	5	1	1	1
Total for each database	26	16	18	17

Ranking: 5 = excellent, 4 = very good, 3 = average, 2 = fair, 1 = poor.

best decision is no decision or to delay. For difficult decisions, experience, intuition, and judgment may be needed, as well. A decision matrix is a simple tool to organize all the important criteria related to a decision. The criteria are ranked for each alternative and totaled which allows the decision to be made objectively. An example of a decision matrix can be found in Table 11.1 for weighing various transplant databases.

- Plan and organize. Planning and organizing are the cornerstones of good leadership and good management. Without these tools an organization is at the mercy of the current circumstances. With a vision in place and communicated to staff, the next steps are to identify action steps, resources, and obstacles involved in actualizing the vision. Involve other key stakeholders in the process. Set priorities and develop contingencies. Prepare a timeline with milestones. Organize staff and resources around the goals, delegate tasks, and measure progress.

  Also, do not forget to plan for the unexpected events that may occur such as natural disasters and sentinel events. These need to be handled quickly with policies and procedures in place so that all staff knows how to respond. Having a pre-prepared plan of action will mitigate any negative effects on public opinion and restore faith that the organization is on top of the situation.
- Drive results. Leaders understand the importance of achieving corporate objectives, targets, and meeting deadlines in order to advance in the organization. This goes hand in hand with setting reasonable goals, empowering the team to move strategy forward, and motivating the team to achieve exemplary results. Results need to be measured against the strategic plan. When execution of strategy fails, it is usually due to a lack of resources, the wrong people in place, or the misjudgment of challenges or obstacles [11].
- Develop influence. Leaders have presence and authority and they enjoy being in charge. They understand that in order to lead an organization,

it takes more than formal authority—it takes influence. This involves building alliances and supportive networks. This can be accomplished by using a variety of strategies: building coalitions, creating win-win solutions, leveraging power and resources, and appealing to another's interests [12].

Some other developmental tips for becoming a great leader are to find resources that are available in your organization or opportunities in the community. Join your organization's leadership development program, if one exists. This is an excellent way to build skills and network with other future leaders. This will cement those critical relationships necessary to influence cross departmentally. Become a board member of community or professional organizations such as the National Kidney Foundation (NKF), UNOS, American Society of Transplantation (AST), and others. Participate in the UNOS regional conferences or get involved in organ donation. The experience gained will be a launching pad for future success.

It is also important to continue lifelong learning and be aware of current developments in the field. Participate in continuing education, attend seminars, read books, take courses, and pursue advanced degrees. Administrators should acquaint themselves with both the scientific and business aspects of transplantation. Attending patient-selection committee meetings is a good way to begin to learn about the clinical aspects of transplantation. In addition, transplant is a rapidly changing field. To keep up to date, network with others, become involved in transplant-specific online communities, read *Transplant News* (www.transplantnews.com), *UNOS Update* (http://www.unos.org/donation/index.php?topic=unos_update), and Transplant Pro (www.transplantpro.org) which is a UNOS website for transplant professionals providing updates and news about the field.

Finally, the development of "bench strength" is also necessary for a successful transplant program. This primarily is achieved by careful and thoughtful succession planning and leadership development. This effort to ensure continuity is now, more than ever, critical to the transplant enterprise: the transplant workforce is aging, both at the administrative and nursing levels; the environment is turbulent; and loyalty to employers is at an all-time low. It will continue to be increasingly difficult to recruit key positions externally, therefore, cultivating individuals internally makes sense. This will require the development of high performers within the transplant program. What are the steps to groom these potential successors?

First, high performers should be identified. Although the physician and administrative leadership may have a good idea of who these individuals are, it is good to conduct a formal assessment of the talent pool. According to Quint Studer in his book *Hardwiring Excellence*, the first step is to categorize staff as high, middle, or low performers. A high performer can be identified by the following characteristics:

- Open to new ideas and proactive
- Shares the organization's values
- Highly competent
- Positive outlook with a high commitment to the organization
- Ambitious and desires career advancement
- Mentors others and is an example to staff

These high performers should be mentored and developed into future leaders. Middle performers are employees who meet expectations, are reliable, and may be comfortable with the role that they now possess. These employees need additional coaching and development to become high performers. Lastly, low performers should be moved out of the organization if they do not immediately turn their performance around [13]. Mentoring high performers should be a priority for developing the next generation of leaders. This involves delegation of responsibility in order for them to develop skill based on real-life experience. Allow them to participate in meetings, regulatory reviews, QAPI, leadership committees among others. In addition, it is important to allow them to fail. Failure is often a better teacher than success. As confidence and competencies grow, provide promotional opportunities—it is important to retain these high performers. It would be unfortunate if they were mentored and developed for higher-level positions but then recruited away by a competitor.

Succession planning also extends to transplant physicians and surgeons in order to maintain continuity of operations from both an operational and regulatory standpoint. UNOS requires transplant programs to have qualified key personnel in place at all times. Therefore, it is important for programs to have additional surgeons and physicians on staff who could meet the OPTN primary surgeon/physician criteria in order to provide a smooth transition if there were any unplanned or planned departures. Ways to accomplish this might be

- maintaining enough involvement in the transplant program to acquire sufficient transplant and procurement experience (for surgeons) or patient care experience (for physicians);
- maintaining current working knowledge by actively participating in all aspects of transplant patient care, including performing transplants and procurements (for surgeons) [14].

In conclusion, as one looks into the future of transplantation, there are promises and pitfalls: the promise of new technology such as xenotransplantation and regenerative medicine; and the pitfalls of a shrinking organ supply and increased regulatory scrutiny which diminishes innovation and consolidates the number of OPOs and transplant centers. Transplantation has always been an exciting and challenging field and will continue to be so. Leadership will play a pivotal role in shaping the future of the field and maintaining its viability. Recognition goes to those in the transplant community who have had the foresight to develop programs to launch young men and women in the career of transplant administration and to those who are mentoring new leaders. However, more must be done—each of us who has had the privilege to be a part of this field must do their part to support and secure transplantation for the future.

References

1 Covey S. *The Seven Habits of Highly Effective People*. New York: Simon and Schuster; 1989: 101.
2 Kotter JP. What leaders do. *Harvard Business Review 10 Must Reads*. 2011:38.
3 Kotter JP. What leaders do. *Harvard Business Review 10 Must Reads*. 2011:39.
4 Watkins MD. How managers become leaders. *Harvard Business Review*. June 2012: 4.
5 Goleman D. *Primal Leadership*. Boston, MA: Harvard Business School Press; 2002:55.
6 Goleman D. *Primal Leadership*. Boston, MA: Harvard Business School Press; 2002:85.
7 Goleman D. *Emotional Intelligence*. New York: Bantam Books; 1995:xii.
8 Covey S. *Principle-Centered Leadership*. New York: Fireside; 1990: 18.
9 Hoffman P. Fear of conflict: management and ethical costs. *Healthcare Executive*. 2012;27:58.
10 Smith M. Coaching for organizational success. *Healthcare Executive*. 2012;27:64.
11 Bossidy L, Charan R. *Execution: The Discipline of Getting Things Done*. New York: Crown Business; 2002:7.
12 Gebelein SH, Nelson-Neuhaus KJ, Skube CJ, et al. *Successful Manager's Handbook*. 7th ed. Minneapolis, MN: Personal Decisions International; 2004:158.
13 Studer Q. *Hardwiring Excellence*. Gulf Breeze, FL: Firestarter Publishing; 2003:125.
14 UNOS. 2012 Evaluation Plan (p. 312). http://optn.transplant.hrsa.gov/ContentDocuments/Evaluation_Plan.pdf. Accessed October 14, 2013.

APPENDIX 1

Human Resources: Lists of Transplant Staff Duties

Pre-transplant coordinator duties:

- Identifies and evaluates the health status of patients in need of kidney and/or pancreas transplant.
- Coordinates pretransplant work-up and evaluation for deceased and living donor transplants. Enters all nursing documentation including test results into transplant database and/or medical record.
- Assumes on-call responsibility (24 hours per day) to coordinate acceptance and procurement of organs with the transplant surgeon through UNet.
- Completes nursing assessment on all new transplant candidates and donors maintain medical records for donors and patients in active caseload following established protocol.
- Communicates assessment data and findings to other members of the transplant team.
- Coordinates all aspects of pretransplant and living donor education program as assigned.
- Takes a lead role in transplant meetings, voicing opinions, and problem solving as appropriate.
- Provides ongoing in-services and continuing education programs on transplantation to other healthcare professionals, patients, and members of the community.
- Ensures that histocompatibility testing, antibody screening, and other pertinent tests are performed for all potential transplant patients and/or living donors.
- Maintains and publishes active waiting list regularly to referring centers.
- Participates in the development of policies and procedures of the department.
- Perform waitlist management of patients ensuring that all patients are appropriately listed and ready for transplant.
- Acts as a liaison between the program and UNOS. Completes necessary documentation for tissue typing, candidate listing, and crossmatching through UNOS as appropriate.

Transplant Administration, First Edition. Edited by Lisa Norris.

Companion website: www.wiley.com/go/norris/transplantadmin

- Participates in and contributes to quality assurance and improvement programs.
- Completes all relevant UNOS forms through UNet in a timely manner.
- Appropriately prepares and presents cases to selection committee and completes follow-up actions as indicated.
- Takes call to coordinate the transplant surgery and to deal with patient mergencies.
- Completes review of entire caseload at least annually, initiating appropriate contact with the patient and documenting actions.
- Conducts onsite visits with dialysis centers for staff and patient education/evaluations.

Post-transplant coordinator duties:

- Assesses post-transplant patient needs, including physical, psychosocial, and educational in the transplant clinic.
- Revises assessment in keeping with patient's progress.
- Documents nursing assessment and interventions utilizing patient care summary, progress notes, and nursing assessment tools.
- Enters diagnosis, actions, and medications in database on all patients. Is responsible for updating data at each visit to reflect updated information.
- Provides direct nursing care to patients in the clinic following established policies and procedures.
- Provides education to patients and their families regarding medication, post-transplant care, and discharge instructions for patients in the unit.
- Manages unexpected clinic walk-in patients efficiently and effectively.
- Reviews all patients' laboratory results, make appropriate judgements, and discusses data with physician and/or nurse practitioner.
- Manages caseload effectively by ensuring all follow-up care is communicated to patients regarding medications, treatments, and changes in plan of care.
- Responds to all incoming calls from external customers appropriately. Effectively manages follow-up care on the telephone with patients.
- Responds to patient requests for medication refills in a quick and efficient manner.
- Assists with scheduling of patient procedures, admissions, and tests.
- Enters all appropriate patient data into the Unet system and transplant database.
- Effectively oversees the assistants and support staff in the clinical setting, reporting problems appropriately to the clinical manager. This may include desk coverage whenever necessary.
- Assists clinical manager and transplant team in problem solving and managing patient care. Acts as liaison between the patient and physician.

- May participate in studies and research projects as an active member of the transplant team.
- Participates in multi-disciplinary patient care conferences and ensures that there is appropriate hand offs from the in-patient coordinator so that there is continuity in patient care.
- Participates in and contributes to quality assurance and improvement programs of the transplant program.
- Assists clinical manager, other transplant coordinators, and team members as needed.
- Takes call to deal with post-transplant patient emergencies.
- Enters all appropriate and necessary patient data into the UNet system and transplant database in a timely manner.

In-patient transplant coordinator duties:

- Acting as part of the multidisciplinary transplant team, the in-patient transplant coordinator identifies the health status and nursing care needs of renal and pancreas transplant patients, living donors, and families.
- Identifies and evaluates patient and family learning needs including ability and readiness to learn. Provides education regarding post-transplant care and follow-up. Documents appropriately.
- Monitors ongoing plan of care through daily rounding and charge review and implements changes accordingly. Identifies adverse changes in patient's status and assumes reasonability for implementing corrective plan of action.
- Organizes and participates in patient care conferences.
- Identifies patient need for collaborative resources with multidisciplinary team, i.e., social services, dietitian, case management, etc. Assesses the needs for follow-up care after discharge and makes appropriate referrals including ordering transplant medications for discharge home.
- Assesses quality of nursing care delivered on unit and identifies areas requiring improvement. Works with nurse manager to implement corrective plan of action.
- Identifies staff education needs and collaborates with nurse manager/nursing education to implement educational programs including the provision of in-service education and orientation to new and existing staff.
- Assists and provides instruction to nursing staff regarding nursing care for transplant patients requiring specialized procedures.
- Serves as a consultant with clinical expertise in transplantation, to nursing staff and other departments (ICU, PACU, etc.) within the institution as indicated.
- Provides current literature, articles, professional journals, and research reports in specialized area of clinical expertise for nursing personnel.

- Responsible for informing the referring dialysis unit/referring nephrologist of the patient's clinical status immediately post-transplant.
- Responsible for tracking and entering clinical data for in-patient hospitalizations for all transplant patients. Maintains patient flow sheets and enters pertinent information into database including discharge summaries.
- Responsible for follow-up contact of all new and readmitted transplant patients and living donors within 24 hours to 1 week of discharge home.
- Provides coverage to the transplant clinic as necessary. Able to perform nursing assessment, direct nursing care, and appropriate documentation to post-transplant patients in these settings following established policies and procedures.

Administrative director duties:

- Consults with medical directors and the Vice President in the development, implementation, and administration of policies and procedures to achieve short- and long-range goals and objectives for all programs.
- Develops and secures the approval of the annual operating personnel and capital budgets. Monitors and explains variances for monthly responsibility reports.
- Interviews, hires, counsels, evaluates, and recommends termination of assigned personnel.
- Develops and operationalize transplant programs by
    - advising the hospital on program changes;
    - benchmarking programs with national or internal standards;
    - working with physicians associated with the program to establish protocols;
    - coordinating the implementation and evaluation of special procedures and testing with other departments;
    - tracking and evaluating reimbursement information;
    - monitoring programs to ensure successful implementation and recommend modifications as required.
- Develops and coordinates the implementation of marketing plans to meet the goals and objectives of the transplant programs. Develops brochures and written materials, coordinates the development of displays and exhibits, and attends conventions and conferences to market programs.
- In conjuction with key stakeholders, develops and executes strategic plan taking into account the mission and vision statements of the transplant program and the hospital.
- Designs and carries out quality improvement programs. Ensures that assigned departments are in compliance with all accrediting regulatory

agency standards, policies, and procedures defined by hospital. Ensures departmental adherence to regulations governing end-stage renal disease, TJC, UNOS and CMS. Coordinates onsite surveys as needed.
- Identifies educational needs of departments supporting the transplant programs and recommends, provides, and/or facilitates in-service programs to increase awareness of transplant programs, policies, procedures, and other pertinent information.
- Develops and maintains cooperative working relationships with physicians, departments, community organizations, and other healthcare facilities in order to gather and exchange information, develop and implement solutions to problems, and ensure growth and the programs.
- Serves as liaison with professional and community organizations by serving on boards and committees, attending meetings, making presentations, and participating in other activities as required.
- Ensures consistent and accurate documentation of programs and patient data between hospital and external organizations involved in the transplant network (i.e., UNOS and OPO).
- Designs, operationalizes, and evaluates clinical and financial managed care agreements with insurance providers.
- Ensures the maintenance of licensure and employee files for all the staff.
- Maintains and ensures confidentiality regarding patient visits, medical information, other employees, and clinical business.

Clinical manager duties:
- Supervises and directs clinical and clinical support staff, including participation in the hiring and performance management/review process.
- Participates in the development and implementation of performance improvement activities, ensuring that clinical and operational improvements are achieved.
- Coordinates patient care activities and ensures appropriate data are documented in the medical record and the transplant database. Arranges for clinical services, evaluates clinical data, and triages clinical questions/concerns to appropriate members of the multi-disciplinary team.
- Develops, coordinates, implements, and evaluates educational programs for patients including pretransplant, in-patient, and post-transplant education.
- Ensures nursing compliance with regulatory requirements, including TJC, DHS, UNOS, and CMS.
- Develops, coordinates, and implements continuing education programs for staff.
- Coordinates, in conjunction with the transplant liaison, community education and outreach.

- Demonstrates leadership.
  - Copes with stress and change positively.
  - Coaches clinical staff to develop skills and knowledge.
  - Promotes safe work practices among staff to prevent injuries to employees and others.
  - Can effectively manage multiple priorities/processes as evidenced by projects and targets met in a timely manner.
  - Demonstrates the ability to translate hospital vision/mission to the team.
  - Demonstrates the ability to set realistic goals for each program and implements plans effectively.
  - Demonstrates the ability to maintain effective teams.
  - Provides leadership to program to meet or exceed internal and external customer expectations as evidenced by patient and associate satisfaction scores.

Financial coordinator duties:

- Obtains detailed patient insurance benefit information for all aspects for the transplant process, including, but not limited to, outpatient drugs, organ acquisition, follow-up clinic visits, travel, and housing, if necessary.
- Discusses benefits and other transplant financial issues with patients and/or family members during the initial evaluation.
- Advises patients on insurance and billing issues and options. Serves as a resource for patients and their family members on financial matters.
- Obtains all necessary payor authorizations. Verifies transplant coverage and other medical benefits and acquires necessary referrals and authorizations.
- Communicates appropriately to transplant coordinator and social services regarding potential approval of patients.
- Assists with in-patient and outpatient admissions and financial clearances to ensure smooth admission to facilities.
- Assists in the creation of new accounts for patients within the system/ transplantation database by entering demographics and financial information.
- Monitors and updates information regarding insurance data, physician authorizations, and preferred providers and documents data.
- Works with reimbursement department and patient billing department to "flag" transplant patient accounts for cost reporting purposes.
- Works in conjunction with and trains clinic receptionist/clerk to obtain preauthorization numbers for outpatient visits/procedures. Coordinates with Business Office for co-pay collection. Follows up with Patient Financial Services the process of patient billing and reimbursement under direction of the transplant administrator.

- Attends routinely all patient selection multidisciplinary conferences to provide updates regarding financial clearances on patients to be listed or currently are on the listed awaiting organ transplantation.
- Provides reports as directed.
- Interfaces with and coordinates efforts of admissions, business office, medical records, financial services, social services, and risk management as it relates to the transplant intake function and financial clearances.
- Consults with and provides information as requested to managed care organizations. Releases copy of patients' medical records to insurance carriers, referring MDs, and dialysis units as appropriate when patients are listed on the UNOS waiting list.
- Maintains strict confidentiality with patient information.
- Actively participates in transplant financial educational events.
- Performs other duties as assigned.

Transplant social worker duties:

- Performs psychosocial assessment and psychosocial diagnosis of living donors and transplant recipients pre- and post-transplant.
- Performs psychosocial interventions, treatment planning, implementation, and coordination.
- May perform psychotherapy and/or counseling on issues related to
    - adjustment to disability and chronic illness;
    - adjustment to machine dependency;
    - adjustment to life-threatening or terminal illness;
    - end-of-life care;
    - adherence to one's medical treatment plan;
    - preparation for the waiting period;
    - donors;
    - financial challenges;
    - rehabilitation, including physical, emotional, and social issues.
- Demonstrates competence to perform crisis intervention.
- May perform case planning, case management, resource management, and care planning.
- Is involved in patient advocacy, resource brokering, and information and referral services.
- Demonstrates the ability to do continuity of care planning, including reassessment and evaluation.
- Attends and actively participates in multi-disciplinary patient care meetings.
- Generates documentation which is well organized, comprehensive, and in compliance with the departmental standards in content, format, and timeliness.
- Serves as a consultant and educator to the interdisciplinary team regarding the psychosocial components of illness, disability, and hospitalization.

- May be involved in clinical research and publishing.
- May facilitate support groups for transplant patients and their families.
- Attends social worker peer meetings to augment clinical knowledge.

Quality assurance coordinator duties:

- Participates, contributes, and coordinates the QAPI meetings.
- Reports, monitors, and investigates risk/safety events that occur within the transplant program. Develops and recommends corrective action, to improve patient quality and safety when undesirable patterns are identified. Active participant in root-cause analysis of sentinel events that occur within the transplant program.
- Communicates transplant-related quality outcomes, safety issues, and regulatory issues to appropriate staff within the transplant program, other clinical areas involved in the care of transplant patients, and appropriate regulatory agencies.
- Ensures regulatory readiness of the transplant program infrastructure and staff members for the following accrediting agencies: Joint Commission (TJC), Centers for Medicare and Medicaid (CMS), and United Network for Organ Sharing (UNOS).
- Routinely reviews federal organ transplantation regulations.
- Routinely reviews SRTR data.
- May create departmental policies in collaboration with transplant administration.
- Coordinates and implements quality initiatives.
- Completes audits as needed to assess compliance.
- Revises documentation forms and consent forms as indicated.
- Responsible for maintaining the OPTN data entry system for transplant centers (UNet).
- Responsible for accurately reporting all graft losses and patient deaths via UNet in a timely manner.

Transplant pharmacist duties:

- Evaluates, monitors, and modifies drug therapies
- Obtains pretransplant medication history including allergies, prescription medications, and use of any over-the-counter or herbal/nutritional supplement products.
- Participates in multidisciplinary rounds and transplant clinic.
- Monitors drug therapy to evaluate appropriateness of use, dose, dosage form, regimen, route, therapeutic duplication, and drug interactions.
- Prevents, detects, monitors, documents, and reports adverse drug reactions and medication errors.
- Educates transplant patients and their family on transplant medications and adherence to regimens.
- Provides drug information for all members of the transplant team.

- Performs periodic medication review and education on as-needed basis.
- Promotes the use of the formulary by converting non-formulary orders to formulary when possible, but coordinates procurement of non-formulary drugs when necessary.
- Maintains and updates a patient profile with demographics, diagnosis, allergies, and current medications.
- Reconciles home medications for admitted patients.
- Facilitates discharge for transplant patients.
- Anticipates discharge date and medications.
- Counsels patients on discharge medications as necessary.
- Facilitates discharge planning and smooth transition to alternate site of care or the outpatient pharmacy.
- Assesses insurance drug coverage well in advance of discharge and assists in preauthorization for medications.
- Follows patients listed but not yet transplanted to optimize pharmacologic therapy with regard to comorbid conditions.
- Reviews transplant medication orders for accuracy and appropriateness.
- Identifies and implements drug therapy where positive pharmacoeconomic impact could be achieved.
- Facilitates investigational drug studies.
- Participates in committees as needed.

APPENDIX 2

Human Resources: Medical/Surgical Director Job Description

Duties and responsibilities

Clinical duties

This position will be devoted to clinical care of patients who are referred for evaluation and management during the pre-, peri-, and post transplant phases. Management of immunosuppression and complications in transplant patients will also be required.

Administrative duties of the medical/surgical director of the program will include, but not limited to,

1 Multidisciplinary Team Development
  a Implement a multidisciplinary approach to all aspects of transplant patient care including patient rounds, selection committee meetings, and clinics.
  b Conduct meetings and discussions to ensure satisfactory patient outcomes on,
    i Organ procurement, turn down rates, etc.
    ii Candidate and living donor selection
    iii Living donor management
    iv New modalities of care
    v New technologies
    vi Post-transplant management
2 Communication Process
  a Develop effective communication processes for outpatient and inpatient venues as well as between practice sites.
  b Create, modify or review protocols for candidate selection and recipient management.
  c Develop and implement processes for collaborative community post-transplant management.
  d Follow hospital chain of command in bringing issues forward when there are issues and concerns expressed by referring physicians regarding staff or operations.

Transplant Administration, First Edition. Edited by Lisa Norris.

Companion website: www.wiley.com/go/norris/transplantadmin

- **e** Promote staff and patient satisfaction with physicians, facility, and administration.

3 Training and Education
- **a** Educate transplant coordinators and floor nursing staff about transplant-specific issues.
- **b** Develop regular education opportunities for intensivists, ICU, step-down, and mid-level providers.
- **c** Active participation in UNOS regional meetings and become involved in policy as it affects center and service area.
- **d** Assist organ procurement organization in resolving any hospital-related issues.

4 Market Growth and Development
- **a** Assist hospital administration to develop and directly market the transplant program.
- **b** Meet with referring physicians on a periodic basis to ensure physician satisfaction with the program.
- **c** Identify new opportunities to develop referrals and to improve access.
- **d** Conduct outreach clinics and other community activities to promote program.
- **e** Increase awareness of the transplant program within the hospital system.

5 Quality Assessment and Performance Improvement
- **a** Take the lead in QAPI meetings.
- **b** Identify metrics and benchmarks for measuring program performance and goals.
- **c** Regularly review quality audits and sign off on reports.
- **d** Actively participate in quality performance improvement initiatives.

6 Regulatory
- **a** Assist administrator with necessary and required preparation for any inspection or onsite survey by such agencies as UNOS, CMS, or TJC.
- **b** Have knowledge of CMS and UNOS requirements and help facilitate their implementation and maintenance with staff and all transplant physicians.
- **c** Ensure that all physician time studies are properly submitted in a timely fashion.

7 Staffing
- **a** Responsible for planning and scheduling appropriate physician manpower of the program, evidenced by reasonable response times to patients, families, referring physicians, and payors by program physicians.
- **b** May appoint a qualified designee in his or her absence and informing the hospital of this designee.

8 Planning and Operations

a In conjunction with transplant administrator, preside over program leadership committee and meetings.

b Active participant in the strategic planning process.

c Ensure that program policies and procedures are reviewed and revised as stated by regulatory entities.

d Take leadership role in recommending new technologies, new opportunities, and new markets.

Qualifications

1. Board certified with the training and experience required to fulfill duties above.
2. Member in good standing at hospital.
3. Meets all CMS/UNOS requirements for medical/surgical director.
4. Participates in continuing education in order to maintain current skills and knowledge base.

I agree with the duties and requirements as outlined in this position description and accept the responsibilities described herein:

Signature____________

Date____________

APPENDIX 3

Human Resources: In-Patient Transplant Coordinator Orientation

Performance Criteria		
Date	Initials	
•	•	• Initiate and coordinate inpatient discharge.
○	○	○ Write discharge orders.
○	○	○ Provide follow-up appointment and/or laboratory date.
○	○	○ Print out list of medications.
○	○	○ Enter medication changes in patient's record in transplant database.
○	○	○ Ensure patient has prescriptions for all discharge medications.
○	○	○ Update EMR; check patients' local phone number and address and insurance information.
○	○	○ Notify post-transplant coordinators of date of discharge and provide summary of patient progress and issues.
○	○	○ Make appointment for clinic/labs. Notify clinic coordinator of visit and any treatments.
○	○	○ Act as resource for nursing staff. Instruct nursing staff on discharge procedures.
○	○	○ Contact and consult IV Infusion/Home health as indicated. Coordinate with case manager.

(*continued*)

Transplant Administration, First Edition. Edited by Lisa Norris.

Companion website: www.wiley.com/go/norris/transplantadmin

Performance Criteria		
Date	Initials	
•	•	• Initiate, conduct, and document post-transplant educational session at time of discharge with patient and family. Review patient's care plan to discuss the following:
○	○	○ signs/symptoms of rejection/infection;
○	○	○ medications, side effects, and actions;
○	○	○ follow-up appointments/laboratory work and diagnostic procedures;
○	○	○ diet/exercise;
○	○	○ documentation of vital signs, weights, blood sugars;
○	○	○ obtaining refills;
○	○	○ when and how to call the coordinator;
○	○	○ General health care;
○	○	○ Need for local physician;
○	○	○ Outpatient labs and clinic visits.
•	•	• Obtain and explain educational materials for transplant patient and family to include
○	○	○ view videos;
○	○	○ appropriate transplant booklet;
○	○	○ thermometer, pill box, blood pressure cuff.
•	•	• Document all teaching sessions in electronical medical record.
•	•	• Initiate and participate in monthly continuing education sessions/in services for staff.

		Performance Criteria
Date	Initials	
•	•	• Give report on patient admissions/discharges to post-transplant coordinator and in daily multi-disciplinary meeting.
•	•	• Initiate and contact appropriate consults for inpatient management.
○	○	○ Psych consult
○	○	○ Home health
○	○	○ IV infusion
○	○	○ PICC line placement
○	○	○ In-patient/outpatient pharmacist
○	○	○ Other consultants as needed
○	○	○ Rehab
○	○	○ Dietician
○	○	○ Social work
•	•	• Meet with other continuum of care managers, act as a consultant/resource to clinical nurse educators, residents, nurse practitioners, department heads, and others involved in transplant care.
•	•	• Initiates and coordinates daily inpatient team rounds.
○	○	○ Participate in daily rounds.
○	○	○ Write progress notes daily in electronic medical record.
•	•	• Attend all discharge planning meetings on unit.
•	•	• Complete discharge summary with Med list and send to referring MD with verbal report.
•	•	• Orient with post-transplant coordinators and attend clinic.
•	•	• Orient with pretransplant coordinators and attend clinic.
•	•	• Observe a transplant surgery.

Preceptor Signature______________ Date______________

Orientee signature______________ Date______________

APPENDIX 4

Human Resources: Post-Transplant Coordinator Orientation

Performance Criteria		
Date	Initials	
•	•	• Initiate, attend, and manage outpatient clinic visits.
○	○	○ Obtain clinic schedule each day and review for next day.
○	○	○ Obtain outpatient clinic appointment per physician's order and/or protocol.
○	○	○ Obtain all laboratory data, and vital signs, and enter in electronic medical record.
○	○	○ Schedule consult procedures and laboratory work as ordered by physician.
○	○	○ Arrange for follow-up clinic appointment and laboratory appointments and enter into transplant database, to include annual exams.
○	○	○ Inform administrative staff to enter and/or verify appointments and reconcile facility fees on a daily basis.
○	○	○ Perform nursing assessment.
○	○	○ Call all patients with any medication changes and document all changes in their chart and/or transplant database.
○	○	○ Follow-up on all results and communicate findings to patient and physician and document in chart and/or transplant database.
○	○	○ Ensure notification of admissions office of unscheduled urgent caths/biopsies/clinic visits/labs.
•	•	• Evaluate all outpatient labs and manage medication changes.
○	○	○ Assign appropriate follow-up labs per order or protocol. Document in electronic medical record.
○	○	○ Notify physician of all abnormal laboratory data and make medication changes per their order. Document in electronic medical record.

(continued)

Transplant Administration, First Edition. Edited by Lisa Norris.

Companion website: www.wiley.com/go/norris/transplantadmin

Date	Initials	Performance Criteria
○	○	○ Call all patients with laboratory results and any medication changes and/or instructions.
○	○	○ Learn procedure for patient call backs while in office.
•	•	• Initiate and contact appropriate consults for outpatient management.
○	○	○ Home health
○	○	○ IV infusion
○	○	○ Rehab
○	○	○ In-patient/outpatient pharmacist
○	○	○ Other consultants as directed
•	•	• Obtain clinic notes from all consults and follow-up on any recommended treatments, medications, and further tests.
•	•	• Call in prescriptions and refills as indicated.
•	•	• Obtain results of all outpatient procedures/tests and enter into patient's chart in transplant database.
•	•	• Assess need for follow-up teaching and reinforce teaching during outpatient clinic visits.
•	•	• Initiate learning sessions/in-services for staff.
•	•	• Reinforce in-house transplant education with patient and their family members after discharge to discuss and to include:
○	○	○ signs/symptoms of rejection/infection;
○	○	○ medications, side effects, and actions;
○	○	○ follow-up appointments/laboratory work and diagnostic procedures;
○	○	○ diet/exercise;
○	○	○ documentation of vital signs, weights, and blood sugars;
○	○	○ how to obtain more medications;
○	○	○ when and how to call the coordinator;
○	○	○ general health care;
○	○	○ need for local physician;
○	○	○ clinic routine and physician schedules.

Preceptor Signature ______________________ Date ________________

Orientee Signature ______________________ Date ________________

APPENDIX 5

Human Resources: Pre-Transplant Coordinator Orientation

		Performance Criteria
Date	Initials	
•	•	• Initiate and manage recipient kidney/pancreas/heart/lung evaluation.
•	•	• Enter data into UNet.
•	•	• Manage a patient on the waiting list.
•	•	• Complete evaluation and present to patient selection committee.
•	•	• Review and document selection committee decisions on patients record.
•	•	• Arrange for patient evaluation at outreach clinic(s) when appropriate.
•	•	• Initiates and completes transplant evaluation.
○	○	○ Obtain accurate information. Aggregate and prioritize information.
○	○	○ Review medical records.
○	○	○ Discuss tests/consults needed with physicians.
○	○	○ Coordinate scheduling tests/ consultant's with consultant's offices.
○	○	○ Ensure proper follow through on tests and consults with local MD, nursing staff, and physicians.
○	○	○ Discuss abnormal results with physician and order appropriate tests/consults or refer back to local physician.
○	○	○ Provide feedback/information to local physician/dialysis unit.
•		• Initiates and coordinates living donor workup.
○	○	○ Obtain appropriate patient information.
○	○	○ Begin workup after recipient cleared and donor financially approved
○	○	○ Arrange for ABO and/or HLA typing.
○	○	○ Complete initial screening and donor education.
○	○	○ Complete evaluation and present to patient selection committee.
○	○	○ Inform donor of committee's decision.
○	○	○ Notify transplant surgery to post OR case.
○	○	○ Schedule recipient and donor pre-op and final crossmatch.

(*continued*)

Transplant Administration, First Edition. Edited by Lisa Norris.

Companion website: www.wiley.com/go/norris/transplantadmin

Date	Initials	
•	•	• On-call responsibilities.
○	○	○ Answer text messages within 10 minutes.
○	○	○ Have access to current UNOS patient list
○	○	○ Complete patient call back and all notifications.
○	○	○ Notify on-call attending and transplant floor of final crossmatch results.
○	○	○ Have access to physician on-call schedule.
○	○	○ Triage sick patients to appropriate team member.
•	•	• Contact appropriate consults for evaluations.
•	•	• Obtain all data for evaluations.
•	•	• Know procedure for double organ listing.
•	•	• Notify referring physician of selection committee decision.
•	•	• Ensure contact with referring physician (and local dialysis unit for kidney Tx program) so that they are involved and active in patient's follow-up care.
•	•	• Know how to use appropriate community resources.
•	•	• Coordinate patient notification when patient's name is added or removed from transplant list within 10 business days.
•	•	• Initiate and ensure contact of appropriate consults for kidney donor evaluations.
○	○	○ Nephrology
○	○	○ Surgical
○	○	○ Psychiatry
○	○	○ Anesthesia
○	○	○ Other consultants as directed
•	•	• Attend patient selection conferences and present patient evaulation results for discussion.
○	○	○ Notify patient with results of meeting and inform patient of his/her acceptability for listing.
○	○	○ Enter listing status into UNet.
○	○	○ Initiate procedure for transferring patient to another center's list if needed.
b	○	○ Request physician to contact patient, if patient unacceptable for listing.
•	•	• Orient with post-transplant coordinators and attend clinic for 1 day.
•	•	• Orient with in-patient transplant coordinators for 1 day.
•	•	• Observe a transplant surgery.

Preceptor Signature ______________________ Date________________

Orientee Signature ______________________ Date________________

APPENDIX 6

Human Resources: Transplant Social Work Orientation

In order to progress past orientation, each new social worker must obtain a score of 3 or above on each competency.

1. Social worker demonstrates the ability to provide accurate psychosocial assessments and diagnoses of transplant recipients and living donors.

   1 2 3 4 5

   Minimal Ability Average Ability Excellent Ability

   Comments:

2. Social worker demonstrates the ability to plan and implement effective treatment strategies and interventions for transplant recipients and living donors.

   1 2 3 4 5

   Minimal Ability Average Ability Excellent Ability

   Comments:

3. Social worker demonstrates knowledge of the psychosocial impact of disability, illness, and end-of-life issues when counseling patients and families.

   1 2 3 4 5

   Minimal Ability Average Ability Excellent Ability

   Comments:

4. Social worker demonstrates the ability to provide effective crisis intervention techniques with patients and families.

   1 2 3 4 5

   Minimal Ability Average Ability Excellent Ability

   Comments:

5. Social worker demonstrates the ability to promote patient self-sufficiency and self-determination.

   1 2 3 4 5

   Minimal Ability Average Ability Excellent Ability

   Comments:

6. Social worker demonstrates the ability to provide ongoing education and support related to patient wellness and graft survival.

Transplant Administration, First Edition. Edited by Lisa Norris.

Companion website: www.wiley.com/go/norris/transplantadmin

1 2 3 4 5

Minimal Ability Average Ability Excellent Ability

Comments:

7. Social worker demonstrates the ability to seek interdisciplinary collaboration and consultation when appropriate.

1 2 3 4 5

Minimal Ability Average Ability Excellent Ability

Comments:

8. Social worker demonstrates the ability to work as an effective member of a multidisciplinary team.

1 2 3 4 5

Minimal Ability Average Ability Excellent Ability

Comments:

9. Social worker demonstrates proficiency in all requisite skills and expertise essential for transplant social workers in this practice setting.

1 2 3 4 5

Minimal Ability Average Ability Excellent Ability

Comments:

10. Social worker demonstrates the ability to initiate program and resource development on behalf of patients and families.

1 2 3 4 5

Minimal Ability Average Ability Excellent Ability

Comments:

11. Social worker demonstrates the ability to advocate for patients and families.

1 2 3 4 5

Minimal Ability Average Ability Excellent Ability

Comments:

12. Social worker demonstrates the ability to establish and maintain appropriate boundaries with patients and families.

1 2 3 4 5

Minimal Ability Average Ability Excellent Ability

Comments:

13. Social worker demonstrates the ability to adhere to the highest standards of confidentiality and respect for patient's privacy rights.

1 2 3 4 5

Minimal Ability Average Ability Excellent Ability

Comments:

14. Social worker demonstrates the ability to avoid all actual or potential conflicts of interest.

1 2 3 4 5

Minimal Ability Average Ability Excellent Ability

Comments:

15. Social worker demonstrates the ability to maintain an ethical and professional practice.

1 2 3 4 5

Minimal Ability Average Ability Excellent Ability

Comments:

16. Social worker demonstrates a commitment to engage in a cultural, gender, age, and faith sensitive practice.

1 2 3 4 5

Minimal Ability Average Ability Excellent Ability

Comments:

17. Social worker demonstrates commitment to continuing professional education and development.

1 2 3 4 5

Minimal Ability Average Ability Excellent Ability

Comments:

PRECEPTOR DATE

ORIENTEE DATE

APPENDIX 7

Regulatory and Compliance Issues: Surveyor Worksheet—Organ Transplant Program Quality Assessment and Performance Improvement

Transplant Administration, First Edition. Edited by Lisa Norris.

Companion website: www.wiley.com/go/norris/transplantadmin

Instructions: This worksheet is to be used during the survey to document the evidence obtained by the surveyor. Answer all questions and completely fill in all charts. Do not include any HIPAA sensitive data on this worksheet. Complete one worksheet for each of the hospital's transplant QAPI programs being surveyed. A transplant program may have many different organs under one QAPI program, which would require the completion of only one QAPI Worksheet. If there is more than one transplant QAPI program (i.e. thoracic and abdominal QAPI programs), then more than one QAPI Worksheet will need to be completed. Separate transplant QAPI programs will have their own policies and procedures, staff and processes.

General Program Information

1) Transplant Hospital Name: _____ Transplant Hospital Provider Number: _____ Surveyor Name(s): _____ Survey date(s): _____(mm/dd/yyyy)
2) Types of transplant program(s) covered by this Quality Assessment and Perforance Improvement program

☐ Adult kidney-only	☐ Adult liver	☐ Pediatric heart/lung
☐ Adult pancreas	☐ Adult intestinal and/or multivisceral	☐ Pediatric lung-only
☐ Adult heart-only	☐ Pediatric kidney-only	☐ Pediatric liver
☐ Adult heart-lung	☐ Pediatric pancreas	☐ Pediatric intestinal and/or multivisceral
☐ Adult lung-only	☐ Pediatric heart-only	

Part 1- Policies and Procedures for QAPI Program(s)

Regulation: Transplant centers must develop, implement, and maintain a written, comprehensive, data-driven QAPI program designed to monitor and evaluate performance of all transplantation services, including services provided under contract or arrangement. (X099)

3) a. Transplant hodpital has a written detailed QAPI program with policies and procedures forcused on transplant data and outcomes?
   1 ☐ Yes 2 ☐ No
   b. Is the program implemented? 1 ☐ Yes 2 ☐ No
4) Written QAPI program cover the following:
   a. All organ types? 1 ☐ Yes 2 ☐ No
   b. Is it elsewhere? 1 ☐ Yes 2 ☐ No Where: _____
   c. Who serves on the Transplant QAPI committee? (Check all identified and, if needed, write notes)

1 ☐ Transplant Surgeons_____	7 ☐ Transplant Physicians_____
2 ☐ Director of Transplant _____	8 ☐ Transplant Clinic Nurse _____
3 ☐ Living Donor Advocate _____	9 ☐ Transplant Dietitian _____
4 ☐ Transplant Pharmacist _____	10 ☐ Transplant Social Worker _____
5 ☐ Transplant Coordinators _____	11 ☐ Dedicated QAPI Staff – How many FTEs?_____
6 ☐ Transplant Floor Nurse _____	12 ☐ Other: _____

d. QAPI committee meets (or will meet if the program is not yet implemented)?
1☐ Monthly 2☐ Quarterly 3☐ Annually 4☐ Other _____

e. If there are multiple QAPI committees or quality subgroups, the scope and communication between these groups are defined?
1☐ Yes 2☐ No

f. The process to determine what objective measures the transplant QAPI program will look at on a regular basis. 1☐ Yes 2☐ No _____

g. The process to identify and track performance improvement activities. 1☐ Yes 2☐ No

5) The hospital's QAPI program must cover all areas of the hospital (42 CFR 482.21). Is there a clear linkage between the transplant program's QAPI program and the overall hospital's QAPI program? 1☐ Yes 2☐ No
   a. Describe the level of involvement between the transplant program QAPI and the hospital's QAPI. _____
   b. Describe how the transplant QAPI's information is going up to the hospital's QAPI program. (i.e. meetings, memos, e-mails, reports, etc.) _____
   c. Describe how the hospital's QAPI information is going from the hospital's QAPI program to the transplant QAPI program. _____

Part 2 – Evaluation and Monitoring of the Transplant Program by the QAPI

Regulation: The transplant center's QAPI program must use objective measures to evaluate the center's performance with regard to transplantation activities and outcomes. (X100)

6) Is there evidence (e.g., meeting agendas, presentations, minutes, progress notes) that the QAPI staff and committee members are reviewing and discussing the results of the objective measures? (Please note this is different than a case review of an adverse event.)
   1 ☐ Yes 2☐ No

7) Is there evidence that individuals with authority to make decisions about the transplant program's policies and practices are routinely participating in the QAPI meetings or process? (Check all that apply.)
   1☐ Transplant Director
   2☐ Primary Transplant Surgeon
   3☐ Primary Transplant Physician

Part 3 – Review of Objective Measures: *Transplant Recipients* - **Do the transplant program's objective measures address transplant activities and outcomes throughout the 3 phases of transplantation (pre-transplant, transplant, and post-transplant)?**

Instructions: Document QAPI objective measures for Transplant Recipients on charts below:

- One organ transplant program per column
- Include organ type with sample objective measure
- List one objective measure per transplant phase up to three
- Objective measures are either process or outcome

Transplant Activities/ Process

	Sample of objective measures: Pre-transplant, AKO-Completion of psychosocial evaluation; Transplant, ALO – ABO Verification			
Pre-Transplant				
Transplant				
Post-Transplant				

Patient Outcomes

	Sample of objective measures: Pre-transplant, AKO- Mortality while on Waiting List; Post-Transplant, ALO – Acute Rejection			
Pre-Transplant				
Transplant				
Post-Transplant				

List any measures (either process or outcomes) which were not significant to the Transplant program (e.g. tracking expenditures of surgical suite,; tracking patient satisfaction with the onsite food café):

8). **<u>SUMMARY</u> - IN REVIEWING OBJECTIVE MEASURES FOR TRANSPLANT RECIPIENTS:**

a) Are there benchmarks? If not, how does the program evaluate performance for each objective measure?

b) Is data missing from any of the objective measures? If yes, why?

c) Are there any instances where other survey information (e.g., interviews, records) show something different than what the program is reporting in the objective measures?
d) Is the program measuring what it says it will be measuring and is the list of indicators consistent throughout the QAPI process?

Review of Objective Measures: *Living Donors* - **Do the program's objective measures address transplant activities and outcomes throughout the 3 phases of the donation process (pre-donation, donation, and post-donation)?**

Instructions: Document QAPI objective measures for Living Donors on charts below:

- One organ transplant program per column
- Include organ type with sample objective measure
- List one objective measure per transplant phase
- Objective measures are either process or outcome
- Use "N/A" to indicate the transplant program (AKO, ALI, PKO, PLI) does not use Living Donors

Transplant Program Activities/ Process

	Sample of objective measure: Pre-donation, AKO- Completion of psychosocial evaluation			
Pre-Donation				
Donation				
Post-Donation				

Living Donor Outcomes

	Sample of objective measure: Donation, AKO- Conversion from laparoscopic to open nephrectomy			
Pre-Donation				
Donation				
Post-Donation				

9). **SUMMARY - IN REVIEWING THE OBJECTIVE MEASURES FOR LIVING DONORS:**
a) Are there benchmarks for each objective measure? If not, how does the program evaluate performance?
b) Is data missing from any of the objective measures? If yes, why?
c) Are there any instances where other survey information (e.g., interviews, records) show something different than what the program is reporting in the objective measures?

d) Is the program measuring what it says it will be measuring and is the list of indicators consistent throughout the QAPI process?

Part 4 - Performance Improvement Actions/ Activities and Resolution of Prior Non-Compliance, Complaints and Adverse Events

Regulation: The transplant program must take actions that result in performance improvements and track performance to ensure that improvements are sustained. (X101)

Instructions: Document the transplant program's actions/ activities on the chart below:

- One organ transplant program per row
- Program type indicated by a three letter abbreviation (e.g. AKO for Adult Kidney Only)
- At a minimum complete all boxes/ cells for one row, which indicates a review of one organ transplant program being surveyed
- Space has been provided to indicate a review of seven organ programs

Describe Transplant Program's Actions/ Activities

Program Type	Issue / need for change identified (How? When?)	Tracked as objective measures? (Yes/No)	Was issue analyzed? (Yes/No)	Corrective action items implemented? (Yes/No)	Negative outcomes from delays? (Yes/No) (If Yes, describe.)	Confirm that Corrective Action Fully Implemented	Improvements tracked? (Yes/No) (How?)	Evidence improvement not sustained? (Yes/No)
	How? When?					Forms? Staff Training? P&P?	How?	
	Notes-							
	How? When?					Forms? Staff Training? P&P?	How?	
	Notes-							
	How? When?					Forms? Staff Training? P&P?	How?	
	Notes-							
	How? When?					Forms? Staff Training? P&P?	How?	
	Notes-							
	How? When?					Forms? Staff Training? P&P?	How?	
	Notes-							
	How? When?					Forms? Staff Training? P&P?	How?	

	Notes-							
	How? When?					Forms? Staff Training? P&P?	How?	
	Notes-							

Instructions: Document the resolution of prior non-compliance, complaint or adverse events on the chart below:

- One organ transplant program per row
- Program type indicated by a three letter abbreviation (e.g. AKO for Adult Kidney Only)
- At a minimum complete all boxes/ cells for one row, which indicates a review of the resolution of one prior issue for one program being surveyed
- Space has been provided to indicate a review of the resolutions of seven prior issues for a variety of organ programs being surveyed

Resolution of Prior Non-Compliance, Complaints and Adverse Events

Program Type	SRTR Data/ Patient Care/ Complaint Issues	Tracked as objective measures? (Yes/No)	Was issue analyzed? (Yes/No)	Corrective action items implemented? (Yes/No)	Negative outcomes from delays? (Yes/No) (If Yes, describe.)	Confirm that Corrective Action Fully Implemented	Improvements tracked? (Yes/No) (How?)	Evidence improvement not sustained? (Yes/No)
	SRTR Data					Forms? Staff Training? P&P?	How?	
	Notes-							
						Forms? Staff Training? P&P?	How?	
	Notes-							
	Quality of Care					Forms? Staff Training? P&P?	How?	
	Notes-							
						Forms? Staff Training? P&P?	How?	
	Notes-							
	Substantiated Complaints					Forms? Staff Training? P&P?	How?	
	Notes-							
						Forms? Staff Training? P&P?	How?	
	Notes-							
	Adverse Event (see					Forms?		

	Part 5)					Staff Training? P&P?	How?	
	Notes-							
						Forms? Staff Training? P&P?	How?	
	Notes-							

Part 5 –Transplant Program's Adverse Event Policies/Procedures and Analysis

Regulation: A transplant center must establish and implement written policies to address and document adverse events that occur during any phase of an organ transplantation case. The policies must address at a minimum, the process for the identification, reporting, analysis and prevention of adverse events. (X102) The transplant regulations define an adverse event as: "an untoward, undesirable, and usually unanticipated event that causes death or serious injury, or the risk thereof. As applied to transplant centers, examples of adverse events include (but are not limited to) serious medical complications or death caused by living donation; unintentional transplantation of organs of mismatched blood types; transplantation of organs to unintended recipients; and unintended transmission of infectious disease to a recipient."

10) a. Are there transplant hospital written adverse event policies and procedures specific to transplant? 1☐ Yes 2☐ No
b. Are policies and procedures implemented? 1☐ Yes 2☐ No

11) Does the written adverse event policy address the following:

a. All organ types 1☐ Yes 2☐ No
b. Process for identification of adverse events 1☐ Yes 2☐ No
c. Severity of events that are tracked and analyzed 1☐ Yes 2☐ No
d. Reporting of adverse events
   i. Within the hospital 1☐ Yes 2☐ No
   ii. To the local or state agency 1☐ Yes 2☐ No
   iii. To the Organ Procurement and Transplantation Network 1☐ Yes 2☐ No
   iv. To the Organ Procurement Organization 1☐ Yes 2☐ No
e. Disclosure of adverse events to the patient(s) 1☐ Yes 2☐ No
f. Analysis of the adverse event
   i. How will the event be analyzed 1☐ Yes 2☐ No
   ii. Who is responsible for conducting the review 1☐ Yes 2☐ No
   iii. What types of events will be reviewed and by whom 1☐ Yes 2☐ No
g. Actions taken to prevent of similar adverse events 1☐ Yes 2☐ No

Regulation: The transplant center must conduct a thorough analysis of and document any adverse event. (X103) The transplant center must utilize the analysis to effect changes in the Transplant Center's policies and practices to prevent repeat incidents. (X104)

12) Did the analysis of the adverse event address all appropriate areas (i.e., questions were not left unanswered, no unresolved conflicting information, t findings were explained, and the program considered underlying systems and processes and relevant literature)?
1☐ Yes 2☐ No

Instructions: Using the transplant program's list/ log of transplant adverse events select at least one event to conduct an n-depth review, which entails the review of the patient's medical records, the complete root cause analysis, any recommendations, and all corrective actions. Based on the in-depth review, the surveyor should answer questions 13 through 16 of the QAPI Worksheet.

13) Did the program identify:
1☐ Primary root cause(s)
2☐ Contributing factors to the event
3☐ Potential areas to prevent repeat incidences, or after analysis determined that no opportunities for improvement exist.

14) Did the program thoroughly document all adverse events including:

a.	Specific chronology of the incident	1☐ Yes 2☐ No
b.	Interview with all relevant staff involved	1☐ Yes 2☐ No
c.	Interview with relevant external parties (e.g., OPO, referring physicians)	1☐ Yes 2☐ No
d.	If available, interviews with the transplant patient/living donor	1☐ Yes 2☐ No
e.	Review of all relevant policies and procedures and identification of any variation that occurred	1☐ Yes 2☐ No
f.	Any contextual factors related to the environment (e.g., staff schedules, bed availability, equipment, systems)	1☐ Yes 2☐ No
g.	Rate of occurrence and common factors for the same/similar events	1☐ Yes 2☐ No

15) Did individual(s) with authority to make decisions about the transplant program participate in the analysis of the adverse event?
1☐ Yes 2☐ No

16) Are there specific recommendations/action steps that resulted from the analysis? 1☐ Yes 2☐ No
If not, is there a sound rationale for not making changes? 1☐ Yes 2☐ No

If there are specific recommendations/action steps, refer to Part 4 (page 6) to track implementation of these activities.

Check below the deficiency that will be cited:
☐ X099 QAPI COP
☐ X100 Components of QAPI program
☐ X101 QAPI – actions/tracking to improve & sustain performance
☐ X102 Adverse events
☐ X103 Analysis/Documentation of adverse events
☐ X104 Effect changes to prevent repeat incidents

TRANSPLANT CONDITION OF PARTICIPATION (COP) QUALITY ASSESSMENT AND PERFORMANCE IMPROVEMENT (QAPI) DECISION – MAKING

Consider citing a QAPI **condition- level deficiency** for **any** of the following evidence:

1. There is no transplant specific QAPI
2. There are no QAPI transplant specific policies and procedures
3. Performance issues related to outcomes, volume and substantiated complaints are not addressed by QAPI activities
4. No objective measures or limited to only mortality and morbidity reviews
5. If they have a living donor program and there are no living donor objective measures
6. There are no transplant decision-makers on the QAPI committee/group/council
7. The transplant program has no performance improvement actions/activities
8. There are no transplant specific adverse events policies and procedures
9. There is no analysis or action related to transplant adverse events
10. The transplant program is not following its own policies and procedures for adverse events
11. Majority of outcome measures do not match survey findings

Consider citing QAPI **standard- level deficiency** (SLD) for **any** of the following evidence:

1. Communication about transplant QAPI activities and outcomes is not integrated into the hospital's operations
2. System is not in place and implemented for communicating changes, updates and activities related to transplant QAPI
3. Transplant QAPI policies and procedures are incomplete
4. Performance improvement activities not implemented by the documented date(s)
5. Incomplete transplant adverse events policies and procedures
6. Incomplete transplant adverse events root cause analysis, recommendations or corrective actions
7. Sporadic information about performance data

This document should be used by the survey team during Task 11 – Pre-Exit Conference – to determine if the team has enough evidence to cite the QAPI - COP or SLD.

Source: https://www.cms.gov/Outreach-and-Education/Outreach/OpenDoorForums/downloads/QAPIWorksheet9810.pdf. (Accessed January 7, 2014)

APPENDIX 8

Transplant Finance: Kidney Organ Procurement Rates for 2013

Organ Procurement Organization	Rate ($)
Alabama Organ Center	22,000
Arkansas Reg. Organ Recovery Agency	36,300
Bloodcenter of Wisconsin	31,000
California Transplant Donor Network	34,800
Carolina Organ Procurement Agency	31,200
Center for Donation & Transplant	36,500
Center for Organ Recovery & Education	26,000
Donor Alliance, Inc.	31,800
Donor Network of Arizona	29,000
Gift of Life Donor Program	31,500
Golden State Donor Services	33,000
Indiana Organ Procurement	27,500
Intermountain Organ Recovery System	26,000
Iowa Donor Network	32,500
Kentucky Organ Donor Affiliates	29,000
Lifebanc	31,000
LifeCenter Northwest	35,500
LifeCenter Organ Donor Network	34,000
LifeChoice Donor Services, Inc.	35,000
Life Connection of Ohio	38,000
Lifegift Organ Donation Center	25,000
Lifeline of Ohio Organ Procurement	29,500
Lifeline of Ohio Organ Procurement – Living Non-Related	7,000
Lifelink of Florida	24,800
Lifelink of Georgia	32,000
Lifelink of Puerto Rico	27,000
Lifenet Health	32,800
LifePoint, Inc.	32,000
LifePoint, Inc. – Kidney IAC	3,100
Life Resources Reg. Donor Center	15,900

(continued)

Transplant Administration, First Edition. Edited by Lisa Norris.

Companion website: www.wiley.com/go/norris/transplantadmin

Organ Procurement Organization	Rate ($)
LifeShare Transplant Donor Services of Oklahoma	23,000
LifeSource Upper Midwest Organ Proc. Org., Inc.	33,500
Louisiana Organ Procurement Agency[1]	32,000
Mid-America Transplant Association	28,800
Mid-America Transplant Association – Living Related	5,950
Mid-South Transplant Foundation	29,000
Midwest Transplant Network[2]	32,000
Midwest Transplant Network[4]	5,000
Mississippi Organ Recovery Agency	36,000
Nebraska Organ Retrieval Sys., Inc.[3]	30,000
Nevada Donor Network	29,800
New England Organ Bank	35,700
New Jersey Organ & Tissue Sharing Network	39,000
New Mexico Donor Program	34,000
New York Organ Donor Network	38,000
One Legacy	38,950
Organ Donor Center of Hawaii	37,500
Organ Procurement Agency of Michigan	37,000
Gift of Hope[5]	34,600
Gift of Hope[5] – Living Related	8,700
Southwest Transplant Alliance	34,800
Southwest Transplant Alliance – Paired Living Donor	11,000
Tennessee Donor Services – Living Related	18,000
Tennessee Donor Services	28,000
Texas Organ Sharing Alliance	28,200
Transplant Resource Center of Maryland	33,000
University of Miami Life Alliance	31,000
Upstate New York Transplant Services, Inc.	35,000
Washington Reg. Transplant Community – Living Non-Related	31,950
Washington Reg. Transplant Community	32,680

[1]Perfusion service for living related.	600
[2]Perfusion service for living related.	1,000
[3]Perfusion service for living related.	1,000

[4]Perfusion service for non-directed living non-related.

[5]Formerly Regional Organ Bank of Illinois.

Reference: Cahaba Government Benefit Administrators.

APPENDIX 9

Managed Care Contracting: UNOS RFI Example

2012 Lucile Salter Packard Children's Hospital **Liver Transplant Program**

Part A: General Information

A-1. Accreditation/certification

Medicare	Yes ☑	No ☐	Date: 08/18/2008
OPTN/UNOS	Yes ☑	No ☐	Date: 11/06/1991
Have there been any changes in Medicare or OPTN/UNOS status?	Yes ☑	No ☐	

If yes, please explain.

In March 2009, the Pediatric Liver Transplant program at Lucile Packard Children's Hospital received OPTN approval to be a part of Lucile Packard's OPTN designation of "CAPC" moving forward. Historically, the pediatric liver transplant program was always a part of Stanford Hospital and Clinic's "CASU" designation. However, from 2009 and moving forward, the program will now report and operate independently under a separate and distinct "CAPC" designation with the OPTN.

A-2. Procedures performed since date of first transplant through last calendar year. Includes adult and pediatrics (ages < 18), re-transplants and multi-organ transplants.

Date of first adult transplant:	02/01/1995	Whole Grafts	Volume:	
		Technical Variant Grafts (reduced, split or living donor grafts)	Volume:	
Date of first pediatric transplant:	02/16/1995	Whole Grafts	Volume:	332
		Technical Variant Grafts (reduced, split or living donor grafts)	Volume:	178
Date of first living donor adult transplant:	05/17/2000		Volume:	
Date of first living donor pediatric transplant:	04/21/1995		Volume:	49

A-3. Has the program been closed or suspended for any reason during the program s history? Yes ☐ No ☑

If yes, provide date(s) and explain.

Part B: Protocols

B-1. Describe criteria for patient selection, including indications or contraindications.

Please see attached: Patient Selection Criteria and Evaluation Process for Pediatric Liver Transplant Patients.

B-2. Guidelines/protocols for living donor selection.

Please See attached:
Living Donor Management Policy Pediatric Liver Transplant
Living Donor Selection and Criteria Policy for Pediatric Liver Recipients
Independent Living Donor Advocate Policy Pediatric Kidney and Liver

B-3. Describe center's criteria for rejection identification and treatment.

Please see attached: Indications for Liver Transplant

B-4. Describe pre- and post-transplant support services.

Please see attached: Pre- Post transplant

B-5. Describe pre- and post-transplant patient education.

Please see attached:
Pediatric Liver Transplant Evaluation
Discharge Manual Part 1
Discharge Manual Part 2

Transplant Administration, First Edition. Edited by Lisa Norris.

Companion website: www.wiley.com/go/norris/transplantadmin

2012 Lucile Salter Packard Children's Hospital **Liver Transplant Program**

B-6. Does your program conduct a "Quality of Life" survey that is sent to recipients? Yes ☑ No ☐

B-7. Does your program use a "Patient Satisfaction" survey that is sent to recipients? Yes ☑ No ☐

B-8. Does the program offer bio-artificial liver as a bridge to transplant? Yes ☐ No ☑

If yes, number done in last two calendar years:

If yes, please provide protocol.

B-9. Describe patient safety initiatives.

Lucile Packard Children's Hospital has utilized an electronic medical records which provides structure and control over how health care is delivered. It prevents transcriptions errors, incorrect medication dosing.

B-10. For stand-alone pediatric facilities that perform living donor liver transplants, where is the donor liver resection performed? When performed at a different facility, which facility would report the donor complications?

Donor surgery is performed at Stanford Hospital; UNOS reporting done by the pediatric liver program.

B-11. Please provide a list of research protocols in which transplant patients may be enrolled.

Please see attachment.

2012 Lucile Salter Packard Children's Hospital **Liver Transplant Program**

Part C: Transplant Team

Adult Primary Team Composition

Title Fellowship Location Appointment Date	Name Degrees/Licenses/Board Certification/Specialty Contact Phone #	Yrs exp in Tx	# of tx performed	Yrs exp on team	# of tx performe

This section has been intentionally left blank.

Pediatric Primary Team Composition

Title Fellowship Location Appointment Date	Name Degrees/Licenses/Board Certification/Specialty Contact Phone #	Yrs exp in Tx	# of tx performed	Yrs exp on team	# of tx performe

This section has been intentionally left blank.

2012 Lucile Salter Packard Children's Hospital **Liver Transplant Program**

Part D: Quality

D-1. Describe or attach overview of the transplant program's quality improvement process. What is the relationship or interface between the transplant programs and the hospital QI/QM department? Attach transplant specific QAPI.

The quality improvement program for the transplant programs are reviewed at least quarterly by the transplant program Quality Committee. The transplant program has developed a Transplant Quality dashboard. Examples of some items recently reviewed at the Quality meetings are the following: patient satisfaction data for the transplant clinic and inpatient stay, timeliness of antibiotic administration pre-transplant, readmissions within 48 hours after discharge, surgical site infections, time from admission to start of case, length of stay as benchmarked to other centers. The team also reviews the SRTR data and tracks key recipient characteristics that may impact outcomes if not properly managed. Every 6 months, the quality data from the transplant program is aggregated and presented to the hospital wide Quality Improvement Council (QIC). At this meeting, the transplant program is given feedback and suggestions for improvement by QIC. Key data reviewed at QIC is then reported to the Quality committee for the LPCH Board of Directors.

D-2. Describe actual quality improvements made over the previous year.

Please see attached documents

Part E: Summary

E-1. Describe the program's unique qualities.

The Pediatric Liver Transplant Program at Lucile Packard Children's Hospital is an internationally recognized Center of Excellence, offering the most advanced surgical and therapeutic modalities. One of the largest in the country, we have a long history of transplant innovation and superior outcomes which has contributed to our worldwide reputation as a leader in the field of transplantation. As an international referral center, Packard Children's inter-disciplinary teams have forged significant breakthroughs in pediatric transplantation, resulting in improved survival rates and quality of life for our patients. Many of our patients require transplantation for hepatoblastoma or combined organ transplantation. Our surgeons perform liver only, liver-kidney, liver-heart, and liver-intestine transplants, utilizing whole liver, split liver, reduced size livers and ABO incompatible donors. We also have an active living donor program and expertise in complex liver surgery such as hepatobiliary surgery and surgery for portal hypertension. This broad range of options and the use of novel techniques to increase the donor pool allow us to minimize wait times and to provide children with better chances for a successful transplant. Our dedicated transplant team provides comprehensive child and family-centered care that is the hallmark of Packard Children's.

E-2. Describe initiatives to control costs.

Ultrasound guidelines implemented to change frequency from daily for 5 days, to daily for 2 days. Will trend and report utilization ongoing.

Changed practice from weekly EBV and CMV PCR to monthly and as needed.
Implemented on 1/1. Will trend and report utilization ongoing.

Eliminated utilization of Zenapax. Implemented on 7/1/09. Will trend and report utilization ongoing.

Eliminated utilization of expensive Chem 23 laboratory panel to a more steamlined, cost effective standing order/set of tests designed specifically for Liver and Intestine Transplant patients.

E-3. Provide any other information that you feel is important regarding your program.

Children undergoing organ transplant require life long care. The need for transition reflects the great advances in long term survival of pediatric transplant patients. The benefit of a coordinated transitional care program promotes continuity in the transition from child-centered care to adult-centered care. This practice serves to communicate the reassuring message to the young person and their family that the pediatric and adult teams are working together. The move from pediatric to adult is an essential part of growing up and ensures our patients will bet the best treatment as they grow older.

This purposeful, planned movement of adolescents and young adults to adult care is a unique aspect at

2012 Lucile Salter Packard Children's Hospital **Liver Transplant Program**

Lucile Packard Children's Hospital and the hallmark of a successful transplant program.

Our specialized Teen Clinic is the building block for our successful transitioning program. This monthly clinic provides time for the adolescent to be seen independent of their parents, allows exploration of their own thoughts, and encourages health promotion and opportunities for self-advocacy training. On the same day, a separate support group is held for parents facilitated by our LPCH transplant social workers, so they may be included in the transition process. The Teen Clinic is a multi-disciplinary clinic including, hepatology, child psychiatry, social work and transplant coordinator staff. Only teen patients are scheduled on that day.

Lucile Packard Children's Hospital will not be completing the readmission section in the "Experience Data" section due to the difficulty interpreting these tables. We will be happy to respond to any specific requests for readmission data.

Please note, within the "Experience Data" section, the SRTR donor complication rate is found under Stanford Hospital's OPTN designation of CASU for this particular reporting period.

2012 Lucile Salter Packard Children's Hospital **Liver Transplant Program**

Part F: Experience Data

F-13. Living Donor

Date of Transplant	Number of Living Donors	Ave. Age of Donors	% Donor complications within 6 mos after surgery requiring hospitalization
7/2006 - 6/2007	Provided by SRTR	Provided by SRTR	0%
7/2007 - 6/2008	Provided by SRTR	Provided by SRTR	0%
7/2008 - 6/2009	Provided by SRTR	Provided by SRTR	0%
7/2009 - 6/2010	Provided by SRTR	Provided by SRTR	0%
7/2010 - 6/2011	Provided by SRTR	Provided by SRTR	0%

F-14. Did the program experience any significant changes in survival rates or other experience outcomes? Yes ☐ No ☑

If yes, please explain.

Source: Lucile Packard Children's Hospital at Stanford. UNOS RFI-Pediatric Liver Program, reproduced with permission.

APPENDIX 10

Managed Care Contracting: Sample Letter to Claims Department

DATE

Payor Name
Address
City, State
Zip Code

Patient Name:	Account Number:
Subscriber Name:	Transplant Type:
Subscriber ID#:	Transplant Date:
□ Pretransplant Period	Global Period Start Date:
□ Transplant Period	Global Period End Date:
□ Post-Transplant Period	Service Date:
Service Date:	

Dear Claims Adjustor:

Please process the attached claim(s) in accordance with your HOSPITAL NAME contractual agreement for Transplant Case Rate related services. The expected amount due is based on the following calculations:

Total Hospital Charges:	$	% of Actual Billed Charges	$
		Case Rate Amount:	$
Total Professional Charges:	$	Stop Loss Threshold of $ = $ @ %:	$
Total Home Pharmacy Charges	$	Donor Procurement Billed: $ Invoice Cost Amount $ + %:	$
Combined Total Charges:	$	LVAD Charge $ @ %:	$
		Per Diem Rate $ **x** Days:	$
		Per Diem Rate $ **x** Days:	$
Less Contractual Allowance:	$	Lesser of Rate @ %:	$
		□ Floor Rate □ Ceiling Rate @ %:	$
Total Amount Due:	$____	Total Amount Due:	$____

Transplant Administration, First Edition. Edited by Lisa Norris.

Companion website: www.wiley.com/go/norris/transplantadmin

According to our contractual agreement, reimbursement is due within 30 days from receipt date. Payment received within contractually agreed timeframe will preserve the above negotiated discounted rate. Payments received after 30 days from receipt is subject to reimbursement at 100% of billed charges plus interest.

Please remit payment to:

Transplant Account Representative
(xxx) xxx-xxxx

APPENDIX 11

Managed Care Contracting: Sample Managed Care Contract

Rate Exhibit

Kidney Transplantation—Adult

A. Hospital Services

1. Pretransplant evaluation (outpatient donor and recipient)
   a. Required outpatient tests performed at hospital not covered by organ acquisition fee, paid according to General Services Agreement
2. Pretransplant maintenance care (with appropriate authorization)
   a. Outpatient care according to General Services Agreement
   b. In-patient care according to General Services Agreement
3. Transplant admission and follow-up care

Includes transplant admission and 60 days of follow-up care post-discharge.

Case rate: $58,000

Reimbursement shall be the lesser of the case rate or sixty-five percent (65%) of billed charges. Sixty percent (60%) of the case rate is due and payable on discharge from the transplant admission.

Primary Stop Loss: If billed charges exceed $116, 000 for the entire case rate period, reimbursement shall be the case rate plus sixty percent (60%) of billed charges which exceed $116,000.

Secondary Stop Loss: If billed charge exceeds $500,000 for the entire case rate period, reimbursement shall be fifty percent (50%) of billed charges in lieu of the case rate and primary stop loss.

Services included in the case rate:

In-patient services, HLA testing, organ acquisition charges, in-patient drugs, blood and blood products, outpatient services for 60 days post

Transplant Administration, First Edition. Edited by Lisa Norris.

Companion website: www.wiley.com/go/norris/transplantadmin

discharge, readmissions during the 60-day post-discharge period, hospital in-patient charges related to any living donor admission.

4. In-patient death prior to transplant or admission not resulting in transplant

When a member is admitted to the hospital for kidney transplantation, but dies prior to receiving the transplant or for medical reasons does not receive a transplant, hospital shall be reimbursed the lesser of the case rates described in Section A.3 or 70% of billed charges.

5. Post-discharge care and other services after the case rate period (day 61 on)
   a. Outpatient care—according to General Services Agreement
   b. In-patient care according to General Services Agreement
   c. Retransplantation—Hospital will be reimbursed as though no other transplant occurred according to Section A.3.

B. Professional Services

1. Pretransplant evaluation (donor and recipient) is included in case rate
2. Pretransplant maintenance care with appropriate authorization reimbursed according to General Services Agreement
3. Transplant admission and follow-up care

Includes transplant admission and 60 days of post-discharge follow-up care.

Case rate: $12,000

Reimbursement shall be the lesser of the case rate or sixty five percent (65%) of billed charges.

Primary Stop Loss: If billed charges exceed $24,000 for the entire case (transplant admission including 60-day post-discharge period), reimbursement shall be the case rate plus 70% of billed charges which exceed $24,000.

Secondary Stop Loss: If billed charges exceed $40,000 for entire case (transplant admission including 60-day post-discharge period), reimbursement shall be 50% of billed charges in lieu of case rate and primary stop loss.

4. In-patient death prior to transplant or admission not resulting in transplant

When a member is admitted to the hospital for kidney transplantation, but dies prior to receiving the transplant or for medical reasons does not receive a transplant, medical group shall be reimbursed the lesser of the case rates described in B.3 or 70% of billed charges.

5. Post-discharge care and other services after the case rate period (day 61 on)

In-patient and outpatient services according to General Services Agreement

Retransplantation—Professional services will be reimbursed according to B.3. Transplant admission and follow-up care will be reimbursed as though no other transplant occurred.

C. Billing and Reimbursement

In cases where the stop loss is reached during the transplant admission, the full case rate and any stop loss associated with the admission is payable at discharge.

In cases where the stop loss is reached during the follow-up period, the balance of the case rate and any additional stop loss reimbursement associated with the follow-up period is payable at the end of the follow-up period.

APPENDIX 12
Insurance Approval Form

Insurance Company Name:
Type: Primary

Patient Name: **MRN :** **Transplant Type :**
Effective : **End Date :**
Subscriber's Name : **Relationship :** **DOB :**

Policy Type : **Policy Number :** **Group Name/Number :**
Insurance Company Pho **Customer Service Rep. :**
Contract Name/Medical Group: **Pre-existing Period:**
Auths Needed for: **Pre-existing Period End Date:**
Services that cannot be completed @SHC:

Claims :	General Precertification :	Transplant Case Management :
Hospital Claims :	Company Name :	Name :
Address :	Address1 :	Phone :
City :	Address2 :	Fax :
State/Zip : /	City :	
Pro Fee Claims :	State :	
Address:	Zip :	
City :	Phone :	
State/Zip : /	Fax :	

GENERAL COVERAGES :

	Deductible	Out of Pocket/SL	Insurance%	Life-Time Max	Comments
In-Patient					
Out-Patient					
Professional					
Ground/Air Transport					

Transplant Coverage

Deductible : **Out-of-Pocket :** **Insurance% :** **Transplant Life-Time Max :**
Consult Auth# : **Consult End Date :**
Eval Auth# : **Begin Eval Date :** **End Eval Date :**
Eval Auth Comments:
Organ Acquisition Benefit :
Comments :
Donor Coverage Comments :

	Agency Name	Phone	Deductible	Out of Pocket	Insurance%	Life Time Max	Comments
Home Supply/Infusion							
Home Health Care							
Cardiac/Pulmonary Rehab							
Psych							

Prescription Coverage **Company Name :** **Phone :**
Co-Pay Generic : **Co-Pay Brand :** **Co-Pay Non-Preferred Brand :**
Deductible : **Out Of Pocket Amt :** **Insurance% :**
Life-Time Max : **Annual Max :** **Immunosup. Cvg :**
Preferred Pharmacy/Comments :

Transplant Administration, First Edition. Edited by Lisa Norris.

Companion website: www.wiley.com/go/norris/transplantadmin

Index

Note: Page numbers followed by *f* and *t* indicate figure and table, respectively.

Transplant Administration, First Edition. Edited by Lisa Norris.

Companion website: www.wiley.com/go/norris/transplantadmin